My Flare Lady –

a handbook for todays (diseased) dame

For Peggy

For the N.H.S

"I am a Woman Phenomenally. Phenomenal Woman, that's me."

- Maya Angelou

"Just stay the way you are and you won't go far wrong"

– Mrs Kathleen Nicholls (a.k.a. Mum)

"Stop interupptin' my grindin'"

-Beyoncé

CONTENTS

Foreword

1. *For Broads Sake!* – lets chat about those unkind comments we receive, on explaining ourselves and that bad habit of apologising for our illnesses

For the Chaps

2. *Remission Impossible?* – positive thinking, inspirational quotes and the glass half-empty effect

For the Chaps

3. *Cure The One That I Want* – on dipping your diseased toes in the dating pond, relationships, and rumpy-pumpy-sexy-times

For the Chaps

4. *A Beautiful Bind* – on body image and how a chronic condition can alter it

For the Chaps

5. *One Sick Pony* – on the anxiety that comes with illness, depression and building up our self-esteem

For the Chaps

6. *I've got the (girl) power* – on the importance of female friendship for our health and happiness and how to maintain it

For the Chaps

7. <u>Red, Red Whine</u> – on 'brain fog', judgement, worries about the future and looking forward

For the Chaps

Acknowledgements

Foreword

Tammy Wynette once sung; "Sometimes it's hard to be a woman".

DAMN RIGHT T-WYN.

And although Tammy was herself sadly plagued by persistent ill health throughout her life, she was of course, singing there about the difficulties women may face in 'standing by' their man during times of romantic hardship and [whispers] infidelity. I'll be focusing a lot more on the former in this book you'll be relieved to hear. Time has moved on and most of the attitudes presented in that famous ballad may have changed, but Tammy's point still stands; it IS hard to be woman.

It's perhaps harder still when you're a woman who also happens to live with chronic illness…

So, in having glanced thus far into a copy of this book, by now I imagine you should have established you're both;

A. a woman, and

B. have a chronic illness – what now?

Well first things first, let's panic! Freak out, and weep and wail! You deserve it! Wallow in misery and let it all out. That's what we gals do, am I right?! Fire your emotions up the flagpole; maybe notify local press on the depth of your misery and misfortune! Post on your Facebook wall and await the onslaught of notifications; upwards of **15** 'likes', a veritable banquet of sad-face emoticons and "Are you OK bbz?" comments in various states of horrific grammar! _Everyone_ must know. How else do we get the attention we so rightly deserve if we don't make ourselves heard? It's a dog eat dog world out there and we need the entirety of the universe to know that we are in **abject despair.** Why is this happening to *me*? What have *I* done to deserve *this*? *Why* are all these dogs eating one another?

Listen, I don't have the answers to *all* of it, I'm just trying to do my best here and I've barely started.

But enough nonsensical rambling, and onto the aim of this tome: it's tough 'being diseased' in the modern world. I want to share with you my experience of being a sickly woman to help you try to thrive despite your illness. To remind you that you are not alone in your suffering and that there is help and support around every corner. My diseased CV includes Crohn's Disease, Arthritis, and countless other chronic illnesses. I also work well on my own as well as in part of a team.

As a fully-fledged female, with over *30 years*' understanding of womanhood, and of doing womanly things and thinking womanly thoughts, I feel I can also speak with some experience on how women 'tick'. Of course you shouldn't just take my word for it; if you need confirmation of my own personal womanliness before you commit to a books' worth of my ramblings, then let me just say that my impressive qualifications include historic knowledge of Barbie and Ken dating back as far as 1986. I'm also the proud owner of a fairly serviceable vagina. As mentioned I've suffered from several chronic illnesses, spanning over two decades. I know, I know, I don't look old enough right?! I hear it *all the time*. I may LOOK like a beautiful and youthful goddess amongst women but inside I *feel* like an 80 year old beautiful goddess amongst women.

I'm just here to try and help.

I'd like to act as your spirit-guide if you will, your sickly hero, here to help you navigate the world. Let me act as your eyes. Do not be afraid, I am with you. I can be your hero. I will kiss away your pain. I will stand by you forever. You can take my breath away.

(Side note: if a doctor says he/she can 'kiss away your pain' they probably aren't medically certified and should be reported to the relevant authorities immediately).

Let us begin!

1. FOR BROAD'S SAKE!

Chronic illness is used as such a 'catch all' phrase these days. It covers a myriad of illnesses, diseases and disabilities. But then couldn't all of those words be used in the same vein? Don't all chronic illnesses 'disable' us in one way or another? Make us feel 'diseased'?

Chronic, as it relates to illness, is defined as *'persisting for a long time or constantly recurring'*. Its meaning is clearly definable but the number and variety of conditions it covers is certainly not finite.

Health, and especially frequently poor health, naturally hits highs and lows. Sometimes those lows last for what can seem like the longest time and we can struggle to see an end to them. This can be hard enough to deal with on your own, but factor in having to communicate your health issues to the outside world and you're faced with a whole new set of complications to deal with. Explaining the intricacies of a medical condition to an outsider can often be intimidating and challenging to say the least; particularly if you are new to it yourself and still lacking in knowledge. When we do discuss our condition with others and don't get the response or reaction we perhaps expect, it can often be quite the setback.

Every so often living with a chronic illness can feel humiliating. Depending on the nature of the condition it can be embarrassing, distressing and complex. It shouldn't be, but it is. Often we don't want to talk about our condition, which is wholly our right, of course, yet sometimes our symptoms make that privilege all but impossible. If it is a 'visible' condition it allows for comment, and that's something we sadly can't control.

So pulling on that thread of the uninvited comment, a certain infuriating phrase that sticks in my head, and has been said to me upwards of 168798782784240 times, (at last count anyway) is:

"There always seems to be something wrong with you…"

This is generally said as an off the cuff, (perhaps feeble attempt at humour?) with a snide undertone. It's often spoken with a question mark at the end of it; as though we are somehow expected to answer to it. It's not really deserving of a question mark in my humble opinion as it's more of a statement of fact. I'm not sure what the relevance of such a question is, other than to remind us that we *are* ill ALL THE TIME. Sadly something we are all too aware of already. The only answer that could be given to such a bizarre poser (and I find it most effective bellowed through a megaphone) is "YES, THERE *IS* ALWAYS SOMETHING WRONG WITH ME: IT'S INCUREABLE". But that method only served to get me thrown out of the library and banned from the local church the last 5 times I used it.

Joking aside, it is phrases such as these that are upsetting to someone with a disability and/or illness for many, MANY, reasons. Let me count the ways. (Seven. There are seven ways).

1. **It implies we are being untruthful about our health problems.**

    If you have to query in a suspicious tone that expects us to answer for an incurable condition then you nail your 'I DON'T BELIEVE YOU' colours firmly to the mast. This funnily enough doesn't make for a comfortable conversation to follow.

2. **It makes us feel like a nuisance.**

    No person who even remotely cares for another person should make them feel this way. Implying we are using our condition for attention or exploiting it for our own gain is just *mean* at the root of it all.

3. **It singles us out.**

    We don't want to be sick, and we certainly don't want to be treated any differently to a 'normal' person. Suggesting we are seeking some end goal other than the best possible health makes us retreat into our shells and that can be increasingly risky for those of us with already wavering mental health.

4. **It makes us feel we are appearing like a hypochondriac**.

Anyone with a chronic illness tends to dislike hypochondriacs intensely. We have to eat, sleep and think about illness *every day*; we don't need to hear you give us chapter and verse on that one time in 1983 you had the measles. Just because you possibly aren't used to hearing people talk honestly about an incurable condition doesn't make it any less true when we do.

5. **It silences us from talking about our illness**.

This is NOT good. We need to talk about our conditions because it allows us to educate, share, unload and learn. The more we remain silent on what we are experiencing the more withdrawn we become and the more ashamed we feel.

6. **It makes us feel embarrassed and ashamed**.

As above: not good. Something we should never allow ourselves to feel. Having an illness is a fact of life, not something we should ever feel shame for. Chronic conditions can get such bad press; we need to be at the forefront of changing that, not being beaten down by uninformed opinions.

7. **It reminds us that THERE IS ALWAYS SOMETHING WRONG WITH US**.

Yes, we *KNOW*.

On the flip side of this ghastly and mildly insensitive coin however, when met with thoughtlessness of this degree, I often try to mentally counter these statements with any positives I can find in them. Easier said than done mind you, especially when you are still clutching a knife to their throat and the police are en route, but if you take a mental (and maybe physical; in the interests of safety) step back, and look hard enough you are bound to find something. So let's throw the negativity over the balcony, crushing it painfully below, causing irrevocable damage, and try that now.

1. Yes there IS always something wrong with me yet I'm still here, being alive alongside you, making me better than you in so, **so** many ways, and that's *excluding* my impressive rack.

2. No, nope, sorry I think that's all I can come up with. Maybe I'm just not a very forgiving person.

The issue with phrases like the aforementioned **"There always seems to be something wrong with you…"** is that, whether intended that way or not, they are simply unkind and simply just so unnecessary. As I'm not (yet) practiced in mind control, I can't stop people *thinking* things like that of course, but I can certainly voice my discomfort when they allow the words to leave their lips. Meaning if you're going to openly say something along those lines to someone with a chronic illness then you should really be prepared for the potentially messy fallout.

What may seem an entirely innocent comment on our condition to you may come across as a not-so-subtle jibe directed at us for reasons we'll have to retreat deeper into paranoia to discover. You see, it's not 'just a joke' when you make another human being feel essentially lesser.

Kindness is *so easy*. It's often found simply in inaction. It's effortless! You can be kind by just not saying that thing you know would be taken badly should the person it's aimed at hear you. Just *don't say it!* It's that simple! You can be kind by taking a moment, just one precious moment, to consider the outcome of your words. If you have an inkling that what you are about to say to another human being may be mean or insulting then just don't say it. NO, you won't receive an award for it, but you also won't receive a black eye, so swings and roundabouts. Think bad thoughts by all means; we *ALL* do that. It's one of the silent joys in life. But in much the same way you wouldn't follow up saying "I'll kill him" with then committing an ACTUAL MURDER, you can think we are lazy (for example), without actually accusing us of being so.

Maybe just consider this: Are you the type of person who deliberately sets out to upset and offend another human being whose only crime is not acting or looking the way you want or expect them to? If you answered yes to that then I hope you find what's missing in your life someday. (See how easy it is to be kind instead of wishing you dead?)

*

When living with chronic illness we not only experience insensitivity on an almost daily basis, but also those infuriating and shaming looks of complete and utter *disgust* when we happen to have a sickly accident in public. When we are sick or dizzy or just generally look like we're whiter than the ice caps and/or we've swallowed a landmine. Those looks you make towards us, despite yourself, and think that we don't notice. But we do; and we *HATE* it. The looks of revulsion you direct at us stay with us for the rest of our day and often beyond. They shame us despite us having nothing to be ashamed of.

To some it would seem that illness should neither be seen nor heard. An impossible feat.

One of the many memorable times this look of disgust has been directed at me personally was when I was sick whilst out walking my dog. Through necessity I'd mustered every last ounce of strength I had to take him outside. But it was all too much; I was badly flaring, very ill and had to dart behind a bush to throw up. A fellow dog-walker witnessed the aftermath of this and looked utterly *repulsed*. She shook her head and looked at me as if I'd just stripped naked and danced the cha-cha at her Grandad's funeral. I *HAD* done that earlier in the day but that's beside the point. The point is she looked as though I'd been 'wrong' to be ill in public. It was offensive to her to have been unwell in her eye-line. As if I should have somehow just 'controlled' myself. She knew nothing of my situation, yet in that moment chose to judge me over exhibiting an ounce of compassion. She may have thought I was hungover, god knows I probably looked like I'd just rolled out of bed after eating a dodgy kebab with a one night stand, but it was her instant judgement that made me want the ground to swallow me up. I was angry, but most of all just intensely embarrassed.

These moments are often commonplace with chronic illness. They don't even have to be behind bushes either! Often they happen in prime sickly real-estate like hospitals! Where we are *expected* to be sick! The above example just illustrates the embarrassment, shame and ANGER we are often made to feel in living with chronic illness… You see these 'moments' sadly happen A LOT with a long-lasting condition. I'm sure you have more than enough of your own to recount, but here are a few from my own (never ending) list of 'embarrassing' moments since I got sick for reference/amusement:

- Stripped down to my bra and pants for an MRI scan and walked into the room only to be reminded it was for my head only so I didn't *actually* need to undress.

- Threw up on a bus rammed full of people directly into my boyfriend's hoodie then stuck my face into it in some vain attempt to hide; in the process covering my face in my own vomit.

- Passed out as soon as a nurses' needle hit my knee bone then promptly threw up all over myself.

- My arthritic knee gave way when I was crossing a main road and I had to direct traffic around me like the worlds laziest lollipop-lady.

- When the tube containing my latest stool sample rolled out of my bag in a hospital waiting room under the chair of an old woman and I was left crawling across lino looking for my own faeces.

I could go on for another 56645451354854 examples but I don't want you all to fall asleep/ burn your toast /lose your erection/whatever, on my account. My point is that having a chronic illness often causes 'embarrassing' moments. Moments you'll undoubtedly laugh about later, but in these moments you'll want the ability to transport yourself to a galaxy far, far away.

As we've established though, mortifying as some of these things can be the main issue is often in *other people* making these moments embarrassing for us. They judge. They look at us with pity, or confusion or even revulsion. They think our illness should be dealt with behind the safety of a hospital-ward curtain, where *our* sickness doesn't have to offend *their* eyes. They have an internal rule book of 'done things' we aren't privy to, and us throwing up in the street/ on a bus/ on them isn't one of them. Well soreeeee for breathing/vomiting on you, didn't realise you were soooo sensitive!!

But what do these think *we* are thinking? I doubt it really occurs to those of the judgemental persuasion, but I'll do my best to clarify anyway.
We mainly feel mortified because they are staring at us like we've just arrived from the Planet Zod, we feel vulnerable because they are looking at us with disgust, and while we are trying to focus on simply putting one foot in front of the other we suddenly find ourselves in the position of trying to consider YOUR feelings. Those of an abject stranger. Then we get ANGRY because IT HAS NOTHING TO DO WITH YOU.

The point I'm clumsily trying to make, is that people with a chronic illness can't always hide away for fear of offending others. We shouldn't ever have to. Bodily functions and 'accidents' happen to everyone, some more than others perhaps, but that's our problem not yours. How much of a Meanie

McMeanerson do you have to be to take offence to someone else's misfortune? Or worse, to revel in the fact that you are better off than us?

So it stands to reason then, that when someone is vulnerable and you don't know the full story, if you can help, then you should. Maybe do that instead of looking on in horror like you've just seen your 15 chins reflected in a puddle. Also maybe be more mature than that last sentence, and try to bear in mind that when unfortunate things happen, we maybe can't help them. Having an invisible illness can be hard for *so* many reasons, please try not to make it harder for us just because it's visible to you every now and then.

Look, its human nature that everyone has an opinion on something and someone. We are all entitled to these opinions of course, but when they are used to insult and hurt other people, (who are perhaps more vulnerable than yourself), it's not big and it's not clever.

*

Women, illness or no illness will always have to bat away opinion and judgement. It's a part of life we cannot ignore, yet we don't always have to like or accept. People make decisions very quickly on what and whom they will tolerate, and as such tolerance levels tend to change when you live day in day out with sickness and disability. For the most part our empathy of others with chronic illness gets as intense as a Shakespearean actor's funeral, but at the other end of the spectrum our patience for nonsensical comments and cruel and outdated opinions dries up quicker than my vagina when I see Noel Edmonds.

It's incredibly difficult to just grin and bear comments that sting and hurt.

You see the 'Grin and Bear It' system is something women have been forced to operate since the dawn of time. Depressing thought isn't it? Now I don't know if this is *entirely* historically accurate, but I'm pretty sure that even cavewomen were told by their employers that their loin cloths were too short on more than one occasion. Not to mention that bit in the Bible about Adam slut-shaming Eve for wearing a leaf two-piece that revealed her midriff. And as we *all* know, Cleopatra couldn't so much as walk past a Pyramid building site without being wolf-whistled and told to, and I quote, "get her asp out for the lads". History aside, even right up to modern-day women are told constantly that we look 'wrong'. We act wrong. We aren't ladylike enough. We're too butch. We're undignified. We aren't polite. We dress too conservatively, or too slutty. We can never quite seem to get it 'right'. Which, let's be honest, is also a pretty impossible feat in itself, considering everyone has a differing opinion on what 'right' should look like. Attractiveness and attitude are subjective; there is no one woman fits all. Thank GOD.

As children we are told little boys 'like us' when they ping our bra straps and trip us up, thus beginning the cycle of feeling we are doing something wrong if we don't graciously accept *being hurt as a compliment*.

As teens we are told by our peers we should be wearing more makeup, we should have boobs, and periods, and sex by a certain age, and if not there is something not quite right with us. We don't *fit in*.

As adult women we are cat-called, groped and discussed as if pieces of meat and expected to laugh it off as 'friendly banter'.

Our media tells us we should look a certain way to be accepted, act a certain way to avoid danger, be 'womanly' or 'feminine' in a way society deems fit. We are attacked, raped and murdered because of 'what we wear'; we are lead to believe *we* are responsible for the horrific acts forced upon *our* bodies; not *the rapist or murderer*.

We are afraid, a great deal of the time.

Often we don't talk about these things because we are ashamed or frightened of the consequences speaking out would have for our jobs, relationships, our families. We are told to keep quiet on the occasions where we so desperately need to speak up.

We spend our lives putting up with things we shouldn't have to put up with for the sake of others; to avoid causing a scene or a confrontation. To avoid feeling singled out. This ongoing issue of imposed female silence is widespread and crosses so many aspects of our lives, from the man talking over you in a meeting to the man who attacks you in a dark alley.

But to a lesser extent, this learned silence can also stop us talking about our illnesses. Perhaps through the same fears I've just mentioned; worries we may lose respect at work or even in our profession, worry about how our condition will affect our relationship or family all rear their head. Whether, subconsciously or not. We generally put our own feelings at the bottom of the priority list. The thing is, when you are told you will be ill for the remainder of your life that feeling hits you tenfold. You suddenly find you *are* singled out against your will. You're the sick partner, the sick daughter, the sick Chandler of your friend group. Could you *BE* anymore sick?!

But with this singling-out comes the rare opportunity to speak-up and educate. You'll find you have unique insights that perhaps your healthy peers do not. You are the Oracle of Illness! Gather round while we tan ourselves under the rays of your wisdom! OK well not quite... but being chronically ill certainly does give you an extra ability to teach others about your condition, should they be prepared to listen. Turn what was once ignorance into knowledge, which, as we all know equals power. It's always important to remember that the more informed you are about your own condition the better equipped you are to clap-back with a retort to an ill-informed comment about it.

*

Now as a sickly woman myself, and I'm sure many of you will relate, when I say that I often feel like every part of my body is redundant. There are days where I struggle to physically get out of bed, and it takes all the strength I can muster just to wash and dress myself. But those are the parts of my life only a select few see; my partner, dog, cat, the doctors and nurses caring for me when I'm in hospital. Not through choice of course, through necessity; I'd rather *no one* had to see me like that, because I'd rather I was healthy enough not to feel like a walking corpse 90% of the day every day, but then that's life. The reason I mention this, is because when people say hurtful things that make me feel worthless or inadequate in relation to my sickly predicament, I try to remember that they are basing these assumptions solely on what they hear and what they can *see*. And where invisible/unseen illnesses are concerned that's really very little.

That doesn't excuse it of course but it does require a lot more communication from us as sufferers in order to make our voices heard, and our issues understood. The trouble with that is that some of us don't *want* to talk about our illness. Again this should ideally be our choice but it doesn't always work out that way. Life doesn't always allow us that luxury.

Your employer for example will often require you to disclose disabilities – as much for their safety as your own. This was for a long time a bug bear of mine; I didn't want to appear weak, less capable than my colleagues, or feel the need to furnish someone who can't properly draft a coherent email with my entire medical history. But being open and transparent when it comes to my illness is something that has become vital for me in order to maintain some semblance of a career. I have to understand that if nothing else my employers need to know the main details of my illness so they can best support me in carrying out my duties (and hopefully not sack me when I'm off sick again and again and again and..).

But this in itself can be traumatic, especially with an ongoing and never ending condition. There are things an employer will want to know, and many of these are impossible to answer. There is no way of providing them with a date as to when you will be 'better' for example, because maybe you won't. Maybe you'll just hit a plateau of constant sickness. Maybe you'll get worse. There's no way of giving them an up to date report exactly when they want it from a consultant/doctor/nurse because these things generally don't happen overnight. Doctors don't commonly work to the same timescales your Boss does so it's very hard to align the two. This can be incredibly frustrating for all concerned; most of all the patients themselves. My Crohn's Disease diagnosis for example took just over a year (relatively quick for most people, sadly) and during that time I almost lost my job twice just due to my inability to give them a definitive answer to "what is ACTUALLY wrong with you?"

*

Post initial diagnosis, 'explaining oneself' should technically become easier but that's not always necessarily the case. Aside from the simple fact that 'normal' people don't *have* to relay every sordid detail of their bodies to all and sundry more regularly than Buzzfeed posts an article.

I certainly found this terrifying at first; the mere idea that another human could hear the intimate details of my intestinal health filled me with abject horror. It didn't occur to me that I would *have* to discuss the details of my condition so openly in order to 'get better' – even less so that I would have to do it in a room where *other people* would hear. Doctors, nurses, *other patients*. OH THE HUMANITY. For a private person, or just someone who values discretion, it can be a bit of a shock to the system; the need for openness and a readiness to share. Factor in to all of this the fact that being chronically ill is EXHAUSTING with a capital X. We spend most of our days thinking/ talking/ experiencing/ *BEING* ill, we don't really want to wax lyrical about every sordid detail on top of just attempting to make it through the preceding 24hrs without being consumed by the sweet relief of death.

One unexpected aside to discussing your illness can be the inevitability that we will often fall into a constant cycle of apologising for ourselves. Apologising for that which is totally out with our control! (I didn't saying it was logical...).

Our illness becomes that socially awkward partner we can't take anywhere for fear he says something racist. We find ourselves apologising for the party we can't attend, the shift we can't make on time, (if at all) and the meal we can't finish. We become steadily more aware of how frustrated our employer, friends and families become, so we make matters worse by trying to force ourselves to take part in things we are unfit for. We keep quiet [there's that phrase again!] about our worsening symptoms in the hope it will appease the people we love. We leave ourselves open to injury and progressing symptoms because we are afraid of the consequences if we don't. We put ourselves in danger for fear of causing offence. What illogically polite creatures we are.

*

Now if you are a healthy person reading this, (why are you reading this? Thanks for being here but why? Are you a masochist?), you may be shaking your head right about now like a funk soul brother, saying that we are playing the martyr; we are putting *ourselves* in these awkward situations for attention, and we are being stupid and paranoid. [As an aside, all of these have been said to me at one point or another]. But let me clarify, we are merely trying to live as best we can. Trying to survive, keep our sickly heads above water, trying to keep our relationships alive and healthy and ENJOY LIFE. Because hard as it may be to believe we are *allowed* to do that!

I know it may seem borderline obscene to someone without a disability, but we don't actually *want* to sit in a cow-print onesie watching repeats of Grey's Anatomy for the remainder of our pointless lives! We actually hanker after the ability to put down the sick bowl, earn a decent living and enjoy spending quality time with the people we love. That's not a crime; it's simply us trying to *live* when every fibre of our being is insisting we down tools and give up. We should never have to apologise for that. Yet we do; over and over and over...

So sticking with this theme of 'apologising' for our illness, let's look at this on a slightly wider scale. Speaking as a female, and a British one at that, apologising is something that comes as second nature to me. I find myself doing it roughly 455965156451345 times a day, for one inevitably pointless reason or another.

- **'Sorry I bumped into you!'** ('Despite that fact that YOU were the one looking down at your phone and I had no humanly way of manoeuvring past you without transforming into the cartoon embodiment of a ghost and letting you drift through my soulless carcass!')

- **'Sorry I am taking a while at this desk at the bank!'** ('But I am at the mercy of the cashier who is busy apologising to her colleague for her behaviour at the works night out who is busy apologising to her for the unfair split over the taxi fare coming home, but I do very much appreciate feeling your every frustrated breath on the back of my neck I'm glad I wore that perfume you like because you can no doubt taste it!')

- **'I'm sorry I was late home!'** ('despite the fact the bus was late then broke down and I had absolutely no control over it whatsoever and can't feel approximately 7 of my toes due to the cold!')

- **'I'm sorry my illness is inconveniencing you'**

Only I'm not. Sorry I'm ill that is. Because much like the bus running late, the cashier at the desk chatting and holding up the queue, and me bumping into you and subsequently punching you to the ground, it's pretty much all out of my control.

I don't want to be unwell any more than I imagine anyone else around me wants me to be. And I can't and won't apologise for it. (Sorry if I'm being presumptuous there by the way, I just assumed you'd want to read on; obviously you don't have to, sorry to jump to conclusions…)

But let's take a small step back here: why do we feel the need to apologise so often in the first place? Where did it begin? And how intrinsically 'British' a thing is it? Do people all over the globe apologise for their every tiny indiscretion quite so readily? What are you looking at me for? I don't have all the answers. Sorry about that I really should have done my research. Apologies…

Let's use the aforementioned illness as an example; it is the theme of this book after all. It's also a topic that's close to my own heart and bowels. Living with chronic illness is TOUGH. It is an uphill challenge and an ever-changing set of experiences you'll learn from on an almost daily basis. Your body is constantly evolving, and be it slowing down and/or changing due to your condition, the human form is one we really have no control over. So why, when we have the endless struggle of sickness to plod through would we in any way feel we should 'apologise' for it?

Well may I suggest, that it might be partly because illness, (especially of the incurable variety), is really kind of *boring* isn't it? Hear me out.

I'm personally often compelled to say sorry because I'm *boring* you. Conversation on the topic of illness is as dull as my wardrobe during Scottish winter, and, much like my wardrobe, often leaves people in that terrifying and awkward 'I don't know what to say…' state.

Well here's a little newsflash; *you don't actually have to 'say' anything*.

I'm chronically ill and even *I* don't often know what to say to someone else in my, or a similar position half the time. That doesn't mean we are necessarily insensitive or thoughtless; it just means we perhaps overthink the situation. We see a problem and want to fix it. We are at a loss because it's an uncomfortable situation and we want out; IMMEDIATELY. We are thrown into an uncomfortable conversational pool without any water-wings and feel like we are instantly sinking.

So, how exactly do we manoeuvre our way through this conversational jungle without being eaten alive?

Well first things first, if we as patients choose to talk to you about our illness, in any more detail than the mere basics, we are actually letting you into a very sacred and oft private, part of ourselves. We are sharing with you intimate details that many of us may generally keep under wraps. Of course many people/patients are more than happy to share every private detail of their condition in gut-churning detail (which let me enlighten you right now - is generally an instant conversational turn off).

Everyone has their own barometer of how much is too much detail in talking about illness.

For my part I've encountered almost every reaction under the sun in response to talking about mine. From the mere mention of the word 'bowel' causing the recipient to look whiter than a polar bear drenched in milk; to the medical professionals who are more than happy to discuss the viscosity of your stool 'til the cows come home from loaning their milk to those polar bears for the purposes of the description in this sentence. Look, I'm well aware this analogy is painfully laboured but don't expect me to *apologise* for it. But I probably will anyway.

Really though, the key is often just in listening. If we choose to talk, just *listen*. You don't really have to say anything. Actions often speak so much louder than words and if you have the ability to listen and show empathy towards another human being it's like shouting "I AM A GREAT PERSON!" from the roof-tops. And you are! Well done Great Person! Although maybe don't *literally* do that because that makes you kind of a Mr/Mrs Big Head and no one likes a Big Head.

*

At the root of it all, as with anyone struggling with poor health, sometimes it's hard for us to talk, and when we feel we are not being listened to; it makes it all the more trying. So because I care about *you* deeply, here are a few hints to help you on your way to conversational bliss:

- **If we want to vent then let us**. It generally doesn't happen too often so don't panic.

- **Stay calm, and think** before you berate us for what you may see as our lack of positivity, it's maybe just realism.

- **That old chestnut** 'if you don't have anything nice to say then keep your mouth shut' has never been more vital than now.

- **Choose your words carefully.** Just common sense really; don't insult or judge.

- **Make yourself aware** of our mental state before diving headfirst into an unnecessary and potentially fraught debate.

- **Don't tip-toe around topics** – we can see right through it; if you are genuinely interested and unsure of an aspect of our condition then it's really OK to ask. In fact we generally relish the opportunity to educate. Try us!

*

Just because we often know what we'd like *you* to say to *us*, doesn't mean that we are all bone fide experts in this chronic illness lark. We often have to take into account what a massive imposition life-long illness has on our own personalities.

We are by no means perfect and should no more be given special treatment than say, Jon Hamm or Queen Elizabeth. We as sufferers often don't consider how much of an impact on 'us' our illness has. When I say 'us', I more specifically refer to our behaviours. Is it possible for personality traits to be learned, changed or perhaps just exacerbated due to living with chronic illness? For me the answer is always a flat YES.

One of the main struggles we may experience is in coming to terms with the fact that our condition(s) are incurable. Treatable for most, yes, but that often goes unheard when the focus is on the incurability of an illness. For me, I understand the mechanics of what must be done to keep me well and *alive*, I grasp the complexities of the surgeries and procedures I must undergo, and I appreciate how little control I have over the whole thing. And how little control I often have over my entire *body*. This fact alone can be an incredibly hard one to come to terms with.

I have, through necessity, become reliant on doctors and nurses to care for me. Not full-time, in-house caring of course, I'm thankfully nowhere near that stage yet. But they are the ones to whom I must turn when things decline, or simply to sustain me. I detest having to live my life reliant upon others and life-saving drugs but therein lies the key phrase; 'life-saving'. That is where the discussion begins and ends. Whether I like it or not, my doctors and nurses are the ones I must call when I am struggling; they are to whom I must turn when my body is physically failing. Giving up aspects of your independence is incredibly challenging but often essential.

I understand too what a pivotal role my loved ones play in my ongoing well-being. This is a two-way street where I must ensure I carefully cultivate my relationships as though they were precious orchids. I mustn't let them wither due to forces out with my control. This alone is often too exhausting just to think about.

Essentially, it's terribly upsetting when you become reliant on other human beings to stay *alive*.

That fact alone can play havoc with a patient's confidence and self-esteem. It can lead to blue moods and even acting out against our illness in some odd sort of teen-style defiance.
Something I consistently try to remind myself of however, (and I'm aware I speak for myself here so don't assume I tar my fellow diseased dames with the same brush), is the importance of not blaming my illness every time I act like a complete and utter horror.
Chronic illness shouldn't be a get-out-clause for excusing bad behaviour. It's vital I mustn't shut out the people I love, or worse, use them as psychological punch bags when I feel sore and angry and frustrated.

Yet still I do, sporadically.

It isn't our fault we are ill, granted, but it also isn't the fault of those around us. It's natural we would look for someone to blame for our sickly misfortune, as we are all programmed to do in any unhappy situation, it's human nature; but it's also a futile exercise. A waste of (sorely needed) energy.

The cycle here spins incessantly; we feel physically awful, get angry and frustrated at our unfair plight, snap at someone we adore, feel beyond awful about it, feel *physically* awful because we've essentially caused a difficult situation and hurt someone we love.
We've stressed ourselves out and exacerbated our own symptoms. SMART.

I'm personally not sure how to break this cycle at times.
I *know* logically I must talk openly about my frustrations and express my anger or sadness or pain, be it through talking, writing, going Jackson Pollock on the living room walls; yet there are always invisible obstacles I place in front of these discussions.
I tell myself I'll look like a hypochondriac, or a bore, or unattractive. I'll tell myself I talk about it *all the time* as it is, so I don't, or shouldn't need to rake this particular muck up over and over again.

Excuses are all these are, not reasons.

I know many people who do tend to use their illnesses as a catch-all excuse. I'm pretty sure they know deep down whatever is wrong with them physically is not the root cause of *everything* bad in their lives, but it's easier to have something to blame isn't it? It eliminates the need for any personal responsibility. Not cool conscience, not cool.

For a short while I must admit I saw my disease as ruining my life. I couldn't see past everything I felt it had robbed me of; the future I'd wanted, my ability to love my body, simply just having *control*.

You see it's easier to focus on all of that when you are angry and afraid. That's the root of it all in my humble opinion; *fear*. Fear of facing up to what is perhaps truly making you unhappy, or fear of trying to move past it. Fear of losing people because we feel worthless at our worst.

I'm more than aware that chronic illness is life-changing.

It doesn't have to change every aspect of 'you' though. It shouldn't make us bitter and hostile. We only allow it to take the upper hand when it makes us unpleasant people to be around.

Just as we shouldn't tolerate people expecting us to be 'apologetic' for the impact *our* illness has on *them*, we also shouldn't make our conditions a scapegoat for the times when our own behaviour leaves a lot to be desired.

Apologise when you have to by all means; just don't apologise for an illness you never asked for.

CHAPS!

Hello boys! Thanks for being here! I know this book is mainly aimed at women but I do so appreciate you popping by. I've left you a few personalised messages throughout to keep you interested, much like that time I started wearing thongs but less painful.

You look great by the way! Have you been working out?! Honestly, you look sooo masculine and virile; like you could impregnate me from 200 yards AND win a fight with any other man in any room regardless of his weight and height simultaneously!

But gentlemen, listen, enough of this flirtatious flattery for now. As I'm sure you'll appreciate, we ladies like to maintain our feminine allure at all times. Our exotic mystery lies in what secrets we hold beneath our prettiest of petticoats; neither of us wants us to reveal everything about ourselves from the moment we make your acquaintance! Think of it, what surprises would be left for our darling husbands on our wedding night if we give everything over to you after a mere 5 pints of Stella and a kebab?

But then what of discussing our illness?

When should we have to tell you, our dearest of paramours? Well, from the first chat-up line I'd wager! We have to let you know straight away how physically disgusting we are to allow you a good enough running head start! We are required <u>by law</u> to admit to our abnormalities to grant you a fair escape. It's only right.

If, and only IF, we manage to chase you fast enough and catch you in our giant husband-net, then we are permitted to date you whether you like it or not. And we know you don't!! But a catch is a catch and if we ladies are lucky enough to net a handsome fish like yourself then you must try your utmost to conceal your disgust.

Hey, I don't make the rules! I'm just a daft woman, as IF I'd have the authority for rule-making! Stick to baby-making, am I right?!

OK great chat later loves! Xo

2. REMISSION IMPOSSIBLE

Let's start as we mean to go on here, in a positive vein. Although a sentence with 'vein' and 'positive' in it isn't generally one commonly spoken amongst the chronically ill. Finding that ever elusive 'good' vein for us is often as exasperating and intangible as coherent conversation post-surgery. This is just another one of the delightful aspects in living that sickly life.

Living with chronic illness and all its little foibles is TOUGH TITTIES let me tell you, and it's important we try to see past that as often as we can. It's vital we take a moment every now and then to appreciate ourselves for just how hard we unwittingly fight *everyday* just to make it through the upcoming 24hrs alive. That may sound like a big pile of grandiose bullshit but it's pretty accurate if you break living with a chronic illness down to its component parts.

Stopping every now and then to appreciate the simple reality that we are actually doing OK at this being a human and being sick lark is good for the soul, and definitely not something we do enough of.

*

I may be cynical, world-weary and OLD, [I 100% am] but having long-term experience of life with a consistent and relentless illness, it's frequently challenging for me to take people seriously when they produce that conversational gem: **"think positive"**.

I'm even physically cringing right now as I type the words. Don't get me wrong, I wholeheartedly appreciate the offer of advice and more so the sentiment behind it, and am well aware that it generally always comes from a place of nothing but care and concern; I've even used it myself towards others as a form of encouragement more than is wholly appropriate. It's just habitually laughable and often infuriating to hear such a phrase on those occasions when you feel like your world/body is falling apart faster than an Elizabeth Taylor marriage. When you feel ill 99.9% of the time; having someone advise you to 'think positive' can come across almost flippant and even borderline offensive. For example, 'yes I know you are slowly dying and your body is rapidly decaying faster than a time-lapse David Attenborough documentary of a spider making a web, but HEY, THINK POSITIVE NEGATIVE-NELLY!'

I've also never been a fan of the idea of 'fighting' an illness either. The phrase itself is vague and counterproductive as far as I'm concerned. For starters I'd bet against myself every time I was put in the ring against something like a chronic illness that *can't* be beaten. If it's incurable then that definition speaks for itself; it's relentless, it has nothing to lose; unlike me. I have a life I quite like, to 'fight' for. I have a mortgage to pay; I *literally* can't afford to give up. Jesus what a depressing thought. Maybe I *should* think positive...

We generally 'fight' our illnesses day in day out just by *existing* against all odds. By living our lives as best we can despite feeling like a reanimated corpse. Living is exhausting. I'm not one for backing down to a fight of course; I once got my gas bill reduced by £10 a month after a mere 16 long months of testy letters and irritable phone calls! I know what you're thinking; *what a badass!* I'm just a humble woman though, I don't want to make the rest of you feel inadequate here, quite the opposite.

Although the phrase, 'fighting an illness' isn't necessarily my bag, it's not the *worst* thing in the world, and it's easy to see why it's so commonly used amongst chronic illness sufferers and outsiders alike. I have no beef with anyone who likes it; I just find the idea of 'fighting' a difficult pill to swallow when I'm already actively swallowing a lot of difficult pills on a daily basis. This suggestion of 'fighting'/'battling' illness, and 'thinking positive' all belongs to the same illogical school of thought – that on the one hand you should fight your way through your days, but on the other you should mentally make some changes to how you approach your condition. I naturally favour the latter of these as it's much more achievable.

For starters I'm pretty sure none of you reading this spending your days lying down to your illness as it is; the majority of us aim for as close to 'normal' lives as we can, so that means we may not 'fight' but we certainly don't accept. We adapt and simply *try our best*, when trying seems impossibly... trying.

*

Without meaning to spread negative thoughts thicker than Nutella on toast, it's important to bear in mind that when you are chronically ill or just decidedly unwell for a protracted period of time, it can be incredibly challenging to maintain that infamous 'positive attitude' we are all advised to strive for. That hallowed state of mind whereby whatever life throws at us we can get through it by merely slapping on a cheesy grin, and a blind faith in our doctors, bodies and ourselves. I don't know about the rest of you, but I find that approach is MUCH easier said than done.

As you may have established by this point, I've personally never been one for the 'it'll all work out in the end!' approach. Over the years in living with various incurable conditions, I've tended to favour *actual medication*, a consistent and workable treatment plan laid out for me by people with medical degrees, over crossing my fingers, toes and titties, sticking on a CD of whale music, burning a few incense sticks and hoping for the best. Not that I don't LOVE whale music, because who doesn't?! And I know they were one of the biggest influences on Mariah Carey's career so I'd *never* bash a whale. Metaphorically, or otherwise.

Although it may be beginning to sound like it, I'm certainly no Negative Nancy. Please don't get me wrong in that respect. I'm a BIG believer in trying to avoid negativity wherever possible; it's something that can certainly compound the stress and upset of any already difficult situation. Hospitals for example are often rife with bile, (and not just of the physical kind); those people you are forced to sleep in a room with who seem desperate to remind you that they are worse off than you at every possible opportunity. They are keen to assure you that nothing is going to get better, like, EVER. They'll advise you on how terrible their condition is, and frighten the life out of newly diagnosed patients with inaccurate horror stories on what's ahead of them.

This isn't big or clever, but it's sadly commonplace. In fact, it can often be a minefield sharing a ward with other women; we are generally conditioned from a very young age to share our intimate moments with one another, therefore where better than a hospital ward in which to wax lyrical unfettered about your problems with a fellow female? Whether the recipient of your ghastly health-tales wants to hear it or not is irrelevant – they're stuck with you. They're your conversational prisoner.

*

I have various friends with chronic illness, who, like me struggle with the idea of 'positivity'. Not to make us sound like the aforementioned nightmare hospital room-mates, but we simply try to be a little more *realistic* about our situations. There isn't anything wrong with this; yet we are often made to feel we are purposely being negative, just for the sake of it, for attention? Perhaps this is suggested because we don't spend our days skipping through meadows, with flowers in our hair, and birds fluttering around our shoulders just because we haven't vomited half of our internal organs out of place in the last 24hrs.

The simple fact of the matter is; being realistic isn't the same as being negative, and it shouldn't be seen as such. Please do not assume if we are gritting our teeth behind our cheesy grin, we are purposely *choosing* to be difficult. Every so often, 'thinking positive' simply isn't productive for us. Putting all our diseased eggs in one blind faith-filled basket can often serve as a frightening reminder that we aren't ever necessarily going to 'get better'.

Chronically ill patients will often set themselves mental goals such as; "After this appointment I'll be sorted…" or "Once I've had my operation I'll be 'better'…" These are generally unspoken promises between us and our illness, unfounded faith, desperate pleas for hope. But in doing so we are often setting ourselves up for a major positivity come-down. When said 'goal' has come and gone and we still feel beyond awful, it can be so disheartening we can slip into anything from an irritable mood to a bout of mild depression.

It may not sound like much of a big deal, but by trying to keep the outcome of these appointments and procedures as realistic as we can, allows us more scope to gain an accurate representation of what's ahead (and avoid major disappointment in the process). Easier said than done I *know*, and I'm not in any way suggesting we shouldn't be hopeful and buoyed when things *do* go well; I'm merely suggesting we keep things in perspective and don't expect too much from the medical professionals straight off the bat.

The thing is, when those around you keep encouraging you to think about the future and how positive it'll surely be when you find yourself in one of your bleakest moments, it can be excruciatingly painful. Pressure to think too far ahead for us can be a major mental stumbling block that fills us with anxiety and dread. Most people with chronic illness struggle to think about tomorrow let alone *months* and *years* down the line. There's also absolutely nothing wrong with that; our priorities are just different to yours and our time may feel that little bit more precious.
But when you are considering suggesting someone with an incurable disease should simply 'think positive'; maybe think twice before venturing down that conversational avenue.

(Oh, quick disclaimer: all of the above advice stands, *unless* you are choosing to tell me to 'Think positive' in the form of a delightful picture of a kitten along with the caption 'THINK PAW-SITIVE!', then you can KEEP THOSE CUTIES COMING!!)

*

'Think positive' is a common bedfellow of **"it could be worse…"** a match made in cliché heaven. Both of these off the cuff comments are essentially meaningless. On the scale of Bad Things Happening there is *always* something 'worse'. Knowing when you have a headache, for example, that someone somewhere is fighting for their life in, say, a terrible war, or risking third degree burns rescuing an infant from a 3storey building fire; well strangely it doesn't miraculously cure said headache. It just makes us feel shitty for mentioning it, and honestly a little bit confused and embarrassed. Well done! A thousand medals to you!

So a helpful suggestion I'd like to put forward would be thus; before spouting 'it could be worse' or its ilk next time, please be kind and take a moment to consider that your insensitivity may the thing that is making matters worse. You may be making a sick person feel foolish and insignificant. You may be coming across as flippant and blasé about our plight and the worst part is that you probably don't even realise it. We all make mistakes in life; just don't pile frustration and judgement on someone who is probably already judging themselves more harshly than you can imagine.

*

Infuriating as it surely is, sometimes I, (and I know some of my chronically ill friends do the same), say this 'it could be worse' gem as a pre-emptive strike of sorts. We have progressively evolved to get in there first; brace ourselves for potential impact and eliminate any impending threats. We are behind enemy lines fighting for our own sanity/flaring temper. Even *with* a pounding headache.

What I mean by this is thus; if we are around someone who is likely to say ***it***, we strike first; letting it be known that yes, we are *very well aware* that things could be worse, but we actually don't need to hear *you* say it. It doesn't help in any way. Neither does you relaying a 'similar' story about how your friend/mother/lover/other lover had a headache and he/she 'just got on with it'. OR how you yourself, suffer from the same condition and yet you seem to manage it so, *soooo* much better than we do. If we had a medal made from the bones of your undoubtedly similarly martyr-like ancestors please believe that we'd give first prize to you, you incredible, selfless, breath-taking idiot.

I jest, (slightly), but I do essentially accept that the likes of 'think positive' *sometimes*, somewhere have a place in the world. Not in mine, but somewhere. Obviously it's understood that language is a subjective thing and there is a time and a place for everything, as I told my Gastro consultant when he started discussing my latest stool sample that time I met him at a funeral.

While I suggest there that there is a place in the world (and in my cold dead heart) for 'think positive' and its ilk, I feel it's important to clarify that I see it found more in those situations where people around you are fond of endless negative dialogue. When it's used for allegedly buoying someone who has an incurable illness, it's very much redundant. Telling someone who has a chronic condition to think positive is like telling someone who is presently in the depths of depression to 'get over it'. It simply doesn't work, and it showcases a profound lack of understanding of mental and physical heath.

There will always be those people who seem intent on seeing the blackness in everything. They are everywhere. If you find yourself around someone who is constantly spewing negativity about anything and everything, and if it hasn't already, it *will* happen; telling them to 'think positive' might be a useful way to make them see that their constant hating is *grating*. The truth is, and it's really pretty simple, if you are one of those people who will end up putting their size 9's in it at every eventuality, it's actually preferable if you don't say anything – just let *us* talk. Here are a couple of important points to remember:

- **Don't wrap yourself up in knots trying to find the right thing to say to someone with chronic illness.** Mainly because you'll most likely never find it. If you feel the need to bring up the subject of our condition then I'd advise you just ask us how we're doing. But be prepared for the fact that we might be initially unwilling to tell you. We don't have to give out every detail of our struggles to you; in much the same way we wouldn't expect you to admit to that sex-dungeon you frequent with your secretary, both scenarios are private and leave us open to embarrassment from those who just don't 'get it'.

- **Be patient and kind.**

Don't verbally force us to see 10miles down the road while we are very much unable to get upright. This just means phrases such as "it will be easier when…" or "just focus on…" are often bitter pills to swallow. We are generally struggling to focus on living in the moment, let alone three years/months/microseconds down the line. That doesn't mean what you are trying to encourage is wrong; it is important we look to the future, but perhaps just pick your moments carefully. Don't push us to achieve more than we know we are capable of in that moment, we'll just set ourselves up for a self-esteem fall when we don't reach a certain goal. We also don't like letting people we love, down. So when you expect an automatic gear change of mood, don't be too disappointed when you don't get it.

- **We are not made of china**.

We won't fall to pieces the minute you say something we deem offensive or unkind. But on that same token, don't expect us not to challenge it. We don't, for the most part expect you to treat us differently just because we are ill. We generally have a huge dislike for feeling singled out. Please don't walk on eggshells around us, don't keep secrets from us for fear of upsetting us. We are strong and capable and need to feel involved in our own lives, and in yours. We are *tired*, and simply do not have the energy for mind-games regardless of how well-indented they may be. So be open, honest and if we are acting like spoilt brats, TELL US. Our heads won't spin round like the girl from The Exorcist. (Much).

The fact of the matter is, and it really is very simple, if you don't have one, (or even if you do) you don't have to wholly understand chronic illness (be it physical or mental). You can't be expected to really, especially if you have little to no previous experience of it. For example, I personally don't understand 'The Kardashians' and 'hummus', but it doesn't mean I'm *completely* intolerant of those for whom these things are part of day to day life. I'm willing to learn, and much as it may confuse and repulse me, if I care for someone enough I'll make an effort to be taught.

Is 'Kardashian' is type of hummus?

*

On the other side of the catchphrase coin, we find the 'inspirational quote'. I've never been one for the 'inspirational' statement; in fact they grate on me something chronic. (Pun intended).

In case you've just been beamed down from an as yet undiscovered planet, what I'm referring to hear are those phrases overused on social media more than Kim Kardashian selfies (see, I DO listen!) People seem to LOVE them. They post them online, paste them on their Facebook (and sometimes *real-life*) walls, give them as embroidered gifts to one another, and they even *tattoo* them onto their bodies.

Now, I'm not one to judge, [I totally am], but it's just not for me. I certainly understand why people would feel an emotional attachment to perhaps a meaningful song-lyric or a beautiful paragraph from their favourite novel, that sort of thing is all wholly acceptable in my judgemental eyes; I even have a few of my own favourites myself. I haven't yet inked them onto my diseased carcass but there's still time. My distaste lies more with those half-baked nonsense quotes made to appease simpletons. I just can't get on board with those.

I suppose the main gripe for me is in these quotes filling up potentially naïve heads with false hope. They are essentially meaningless and even trite, and I don't know about you but I just don't feel 'inspired' reading something that requires a Minion holding a rose in order to illustrate it.

But if you are heretofore unaware of this form of 'inspiration' for chronically ill people strewn across the internet and beyond, let me enlighten you and walk you through some of the best [WORST, absolute WORST].

Consider yourselves INSPIRED!

(Side note: Is 'Minion' a type of hummus?)

1. **"When 'I' is replaced with 'we', even illness becomes wellness"**

This one is painfully clunky and borderline vomit-inducing. It makes me livid that it forces me to read it more than once just to make sure I understand it. I think here we are trying to suggest that when we stick together we can reach 'wellness' (i.e. get healthier?) I'm not sure how that works exactly? Do I assemble a 'squad' a la Taylor Swift or the Avengers to help me manage my illness? Do I need to sew an outfit? Maybe I am to utilise one friend to take my temperature, and one to test my stool, etc.? Any volunteers for that second one? Guys??

Or possibly it suggests something decidedly more profound; that we shouldn't keep our illness to ourselves and share with others in order to improve our mental health. I like that idea better. It's nice, and seems a healthy way to live. Plus I don't have enough non-squeamish friends to cover every aspect of my personal care. Look I don't know guys, maybe it means that maybe it means this I don't know, I'm pretty sure I'm reading too much into it and would be better using my precious time writing Hello Kitty fan fiction. *MORE*, Hello Kitty fan fiction.

2. "You were given this life because you're strong enough to live it"

I beg to differ, mate; I was 'given' this life because my parents downed half a bottle of rum, watched Nine and a Half Weeks and had an 'early night'. (I presume). The preceding shambles my life has been since then is entirely of my own doing. In terms of illness, again no almighty deity chose to grant me an incurable illness, there was no survey done on high to establish who was 'strong enough' to deal with said disease. And if you *somehow* manage to prove me wrong on this one I strongly demand a recount because I'm sorry to disappoint you but I'm chronically ill and I also cry my retinas waterless when I see a cat looking even remotely sad in the street. Case CLOSED.

Again I understand the sentiment behind this phrase here; that you should be proud of your 'strength'. But my issue lies in the idea that it is intended to inspire. All it does is inspire me to delete any friend from my Facebook page within seconds of them quoting it, and very little else to be honest.

3. "Don't cry cos it's over smile cos it happened"

OK so this one is not necessarily an illness-themed quote, but another absolutely despicable use of the English language that I loathe intensely. Again as before I understand the sentiment, it's encouraging us sickly souls to let go of our sadness and focus on what was good about a relationship/thing/cat. But when I've just had my heartbroken by Julio who cheated on me with the maid, 15 call-girls and my great uncle AGAIN, I'm just supposed to smile because it happened and move on?! You're having a laugh?! I've had his face tattooed on to my left butt cheek mate!

4. "It may be stormy now, but it can't rain forever!"

I'm Scottish. Please believe me when I say; IT CAN.

Look, I *know* I'm being a cynical pain in the neck here, and I'm not saying you have to dislike these 'inspirational' quotes as I do; you may enjoy them and/or even feel inspired by them yourselves. That's obviously FINE.

Actually why lie, that's exactly what I'm saying; they are penned by Satan.

I just personally feel that it's more constructive to take inspiration from what *you* achieve and what those around you achieve. We don't need words of so-called wisdom from someone who's appeared on one episode of the X-Factor to help us live our lives. Inspire yourself by proving yourself wrong every day. It might be as simple as getting out of bed; take that as your inspiration, set yourself manageable goals and aim for them. You do most of these epic feats without even thinking about them! Don't waste time and energy beating yourself up when you don't quite make it in whatever you set out to achieve, as in 24hrs you'll always get another shot at it. Never take a rose from a Minion; that sort of thing.

Actually come to think of it I'm actually quite good at this inspirational quote lark myself! I've been denying myself my one true calling!

*

This idea of 'positive thinking' and this endless prerequisite for 'inspiration' is relayed again and again in many situations, namely chronic illness; be it physical or mental. Along similar lines, (and something we'll touch upon in more thrilling detail later), is the awareness that living with a physical disability can have an incredibly detrimental effect on our mental health.

It always seems so utterly bizarre to me that people wouldn't grasp this notion.

Well, I say this, but its only now, after years of living with chronic illness myself that I can say that with a level of confidence and assurance, (maybe even smugness); but pre-diagnosis it's certainly not something I would have remotely considered. I was focused solely on pain and how to *stop* said pain, beyond that not much of anything else at all. I picture it a bit like a see-saw, one thing starts to improve and another takes a dip in unison, never quite reaching an even keel in body and mind. The mere idea then that thinking positively will help cure an incurable illness is abhorrent to me for many, MANY reasons. The foremost of these being it's simply inaccurate. Yes, of course it's a great notion to try and take a positive attitude towards your life with a chronic condition, something I try to do every day, but it becomes harmful when people assume offering these 'think positive' style nuggets up as advice when you are suffering from something as distressing and damaging as depression, for example, is anything other than a terrible idea.

I suppose not having to consider an illness as part of your life allows room for ignorance to slip in. Not having to factor these other... factors in, means it's pretty understandable that people would be unaware of the wider situation. For example I, as a woman, don't have a penis and balls, therefore although I KNOW they exist, I never have to think about how it must feel to be kicked in that region, or to catch one of those bad-boys in your zip-fly. OUCH!!!!! Am I right ladz?! So I suppose as patients, instead of losing our cool and murdering those humans with a lack of awareness of our wider spanning problems to death, we should always try and educate them where possible. A lot less jail time that way I've established.

When trying to briefly explain the complexities of life with chronic illness I often refer to one particular example. We'll call it The 'Flu' Case: think about how miserable you feel when you're loaded with the flu – *horrible* eh? YES! Well imagine if you felt that unwell all day every day to varying degrees – pretty depressing yes? YES! Well that's *our life*. Get it now? YES! It's hard to shake off these negative feelings and "smile" and "think positive" because it often seems there really isn't much to think positively about.

When I'm personally at my lowest ebb I try to consider the good things in my life. Sounds like the world's most inane advice I know, but please bear with me.

I'll try to set myself little attainable, mental goals I can hopefully achieve when I'm feeling a little stronger. Although the difficulty here is in ensuring I'm mentally strong enough to fight against my mind when it wants to discount all of my goals in a fit of temper and frustration. Winning the *'what's the point?!'* battle against yourself is often the hardest.

For me that's often more difficult to manage than other people's responses to my illness; my own inability to battle with my own mind. Not that I don't win from time to time, because I really do! I'm a heavyweight. I'm Arnold mother-hubbarding Schwarzenegger. (*Sometimes*). Inspiring and motivating yourself *despite* an illness is easier said than done.

The difficulty in keeping a positive and hopeful attitude can also be exacerbated by the constant bombardment in the media of 'inspiring' fellow patients. Those people with the same condition as you, who are somehow capable of running marathons, or winning Olympic Gold, or successfully doing 5 squats without needing carried from the gym in a stretcher. These stories CAN be inspiring. They show it's still possible to achieve your dreams, however physically demanding they may be, in the face of illness. Which, of course, is wonderful! But overloading ourselves with these stories of 'inspiration' is often also damaging to perhaps those more impressionable and fragile sufferers. Holding our own achievements up against those Olympic athletes, or Oscar winning actors with the same condition, can make us feel we are perhaps not trying hard enough. Or that we are lazy. It can make us question ourselves and our actions. Or, and often more frustratingly, they give those on the outside the impression that we are not being truthful about the full extent of our ill health. That infamous; 'If *she* can do *that* why can't *you* get out of bed?' effect.

*

Now along the same lines, and you may be shocked to hear it, but I've personally never bought into the whole 'glass half full / empty' analogy. As if it's as simple as breaking down a personality-type based on the contents of a glass of water; if you're an optimist the glass is half full. If you're a pessimist the glass is half empty. I don't want to be pigeonholed into either of those dispositions thank-you very much. I'm neither. *I'm both.* I'm a human woman with a cracking rack. And for the record I don't even *like* water.

Sometimes I am 'optimistic' and able to look at things with hope and positivity. Sometimes I'm pessimistic and able to see only the most negative aspects of anything and everything. Like most human beings. OK, look if I were held at gunpoint and forced to choose one or the other I'd probably have to say I think I'm more of a negative person than I'd particularly like to be. I like to think I look at the positives in life but they are often clouded by my own anxieties and this makes it much harder to think positively. I'd maybe say I'm a realist? But then surely a realist sees things as they think they *should* be? As they actually *are*? I'm not sure such a thing really exists. By the way, why are you holding me at gun-point? That is seriously unnecessary, not to mention illegal.

Let's move on.

One of the reasons I find it so difficult to pin my 'self' down, is because I suppose I don't want to be someone who is easy to pin down. I want to have a full and complex personality. I don't want be defined as an –'ism' or an –'ist'. Definitely not an –'itch'. Everyone wants to be more than just one 'thing'. I suppose like most individuals I want to be exactly that; individual. Someone who is seen as a woman people want to learn about and learn from; someone who can inspire and feel inspired by everything around her; someone who knows all the words to every Bee Gee song but doesn't brag about it cos you know, she's confident in her own abilities and doesn't need your praise and reassurance OK?

If I decide I am 'glass half full' or empty I've chosen how I *should* now behave. I'm not quite ready to accept my lot and ride on into the sweet relief of death *just* yet thank-you very much. I'd much rather constantly move forward; constantly improve. Test myself and push my limits. See what I can achieve and stop letting things hold me back. Accepting we are either a negative or positive person allows for self-introspection, I understand that, but it also allows for laziness. It sanctions you to make excuses for yourself: "Well I'm just a negative person so…"

But it's *hard* not to give in to living your life in a certain way, to avoid the negative side of the road. Like an addiction or any learned behaviour it's so easy to fall back into old habits…

Maybe the answer lies in finding strength – mental strength – to break out of your usual patterns. This can be incredibly difficult when every other part of your body seems to be failing. Focusing on the good things to come in the future can often seem embarrassingly redundant because everything seems so bleak in the present. It's certainly worth trying though. The alternative is miserable and we really don't need more bleakness on our plates when our bodies are already determined to make us live like hard-core Goth's. Let's face it, we are all *tired*. Tired of coping with pain, and exhausted from the effort of just *living* through it all. But lying down to our illness does nothing to improve our state of mind.

I don't refer to literal rest here; (which of course is essential wherever possible). I refer to letting the negative aspects of chronic illness cloud your judgement or sway us into making rash decisions. Don't give in to negative thoughts. Take a step back and consider your position rationally – will you realistically come out the other end of this bad patch unscathed? How can you achieve that? What can you do practically to help yourself? Being mentally proactive can be just as important as the physical.

A few important points to remember when the mental struggles become taller and taller hurdles to jump:

- **Spend time with people who buoy you.**

    Those friends and family who make you feel good about yourself, and are generally able to maintain an optimistic outlook. Those people in your life, if you have them, who radiate positivity and don't flood you with negative thoughts, are really a priceless balm for a stinging soul.

- **Don't overthink things.**

Easier said than done, believe me *I know*. But when we fall into this cycle, its one which can quickly spiral out of control; leaving room for paranoia to creep in and making it increasingly hard to get a grip on our anxiety. Hope is vital when living with incurable illness and when that starts to slip away we begin to retreat into ourselves. Don't waste energy overthinking every potential outcome of a situation and try to focus on the matter at hand. One thing at a time. Breathe in. Breathe out.

- **Be proactive with what you *can* do.**

Instead of focusing on what you can't. If certain plans must change due to illness then so be it; don't weep and wail about missing a date, make plans for the next one without pre-empting everything with a 'what's the point' attitude. One setback is only that; there may be more in the future, in fact it's inevitable, but you'll deal with each as they come. Don't use them as an excuse to wallow in self-pity.

*

A little encouragement in all areas of life goes a long way. From the workplace to the bedroom and everywhere in between, we all need a little praise every now and then. These days, in our sickly lives we hear so many medical professionals seem to advise us we are eating the wrong things, not exercising enough, smoking/drinking/mainlining heroin too often, etc. YAWN. Sometimes it's encouraging to be reassured that we are actually doing the best we can to maintain the best health we can *despite* our seemingly constantly failing bodies.

In any situation, when we are advised we are doing something wrong, or at least that it could be done better, we all deal with it in different ways. If we have insecurities over our own abilities or are generally just an anxious person, being handed a bouquet of criticism can sometimes be hard to accept, regardless of how pretty a ribbon it's tied up in.

I'm personally quite a defensive person, so I often find it hard to accept someone's help - it can sometimes be interpreted by my skewed brain as a slight on my own intelligence, or another notch on the bedpost of my lack of self-belief. But when this 'criticism' comes from health professionals I find myself grasping at their every word like a child for a lollipop or me for Jon Hamm's ankle on a red carpet. It doesn't seem to matter what they say either; they could tell me to "try dabbing some vinegar in your eyes" for a sore foot and I'd still nod aggressively and skip out to buy some over-priced condiment. Of course no doctor has ever advised me to do this, thank-fully, but it's an example of the lengths I go to in my endeavour to 'please' a doctor. Now, even years after my initial diagnosis I still find myself looking to him/her to confirm what a good sickly student I have been. Still striving for that sticker or that lollipop that says I've been a model patient.

"Yes, I tried those tablets, and right to the end of the course, doctor!"

"Yes, I've been doing those exercises every night just like you suggested doctor!"

 "Yes I've been dabbing vinegar in my eyes every morning and have only encountered one near miss on the motorway to date doctor!"

This idea of an eagerness to please our doctors most likely stems from desperation. We are DESPERATE for the solution. We want to help them help us so we can get to the bit where we are 'better'. This is often the *only* reward worth having. They are there to assist us in finding a solution to our condition. Or at the very least to help us live the most 'normal' lives we can. They are generally our most invaluable asset in our quest for chronic harmony. We seek their approval because it normally means we are on the right path. If we follow their instructions (however frustrating and time consuming they may be) we get closer, quicker, to *feeling good.*

But hey, let's not get maudlin here! The encouragement we get from our doctors is the cherry on a wonderful sickly cake! Don't take that flattery for granted! You see, with chronic illness there *IS* so much *good stuff* to look forward too!

Someone *else* to make your dinner and change your sheets when you're in hospital!

Pain relief so potent it'll make you feel like a 'Breaking Bad' extra!

The sweet relief of death when it comes!

All of that *and MORE!*

So let's see a "smile" eh? Think positive….

*

CHAPS!

Hi again guyz! Oh listen, I know you think we should smile more.

I know.

I know this; we all do, because you kindly tell us to 'smile!' when we are serving you drinks at the bar. I know this because you bellow it from your car as we cross the street. I know this because you tell us in no uncertain terms when we are walking past the building site you are most likely working on.

And let me be so bold as to speak for all of womankind here when I say, we are FLATTERED!

As we go about our daily business, hearing you bellow from (dangerously unprofessionally erected) scaffolding, playfully requesting we "GET OUR TITS OUT!" WELL, let me just say it sends us all a flutter, to put it delicately! You, with your hi-vis vest just tight-fitting enough to showcase your ample beer-belly; pie grease dripping like a greasy waterfall down your 5 chins as you charmingly make some sexually suggestive gesture with your plump sausage-esque fingers... I needn't say it I know, but SWOOOOOOON.

I'm sure you don't need me to tell you there is NOTHING we ladies find more attractive.

Personally, I'm in a long term 'relationship', but as I lie next to my partner night after night all I can think of before I close my eyes is that DREAMBOAT in an ill-fitting hard hat who once suggested doing something to my vagina I'm 99.9% sure is physically impossible, as pieces of a corned beef-pastie playfully flew from his lips. I hope one day to see him again, maybe when a new housing development is being built, and of course I'll be ready with my biggest smile and shortest skirt!

Until then I must continue on with this current FAÇADE of happiness.

We all have dreams.

So if you're reading this, my corned beef-pastie dreamboat and somehow don't understand sarcasm;

PLEASE STOP TELLING WOMEN TO SMILE.

Ok love you, bye xo

3. CURE THE ONE THAT I WANT

Now, the chapter we've all been waiting for: LOVE! SEX! MICROWAVE MEALS FOR ONE!

But, before we delve too deeply under the covers of romantic entanglements, unprepared and unsheathed, a quick word of reassurance: I'm telling you here and now, love and romantic relationships don't have to be *any* different for those of us ladies living with chronic illness.

That statement may seem obvious to those of you who've never been ill for longer than it takes to get over last night's hangover, but when you live with a lifelong condition the prospect of shacking up with a potential beau can seem as implausible as a Donald Trump election campaign. Romantic liaisons where one or both parties suffers from an illness is undoubtedly not without its bumps in the road, but then what 'healthy' (pardon the pun), functioning relationship isn't?

So it's easy for me to profess that the age old game of seduction follows much the same rules for those of us with ill-functioning bits; although admittedly it may occasionally be a little more difficult for us to garner the courage to involve ourselves in dating, intercourse or even being taken up the… aisle. That's primarily because the anxiety caused by illness can often be border-line unmanageable. This is not a fun prospect when we add meeting someone new into our sickly mix. For some, our illness is the elephant in the room, that photo of us with a perm in our parents living-room; the thing we are afraid to talk about, and certainly don't want to have to share with a potential lover.

Listen, for anyone who's tried to get an elephant out of a semi-detached bungalow you'll know from experience, it's no easy feat.

But putting elephants to one side for a moment (again a physical challenge of epic proportions, I mean where do you even store them?!), let's come back to that idea of blossoming love with a chronic illness. When talking romance, some phrases from chronically ill women I've heard over the years are that they feel 'less of a woman' and 'unworthy of love' from time to time. This has been from both women in long term relationships and brand new courtships.

Of course, neither of these statements is in any universe *true*, and they may sound overly dramatic to those of you who've never been ill for longer than a week, but they are accurate states of mind which can buzz away at us like wasps round your Gran's jam sandwich. These feelings can be incredibly hard to simply brush aside. Much like that pesky wasp, they can get more intense the more you try to shoo them away. Honestly lads, leave my Gran ALONE.

*

These feelings that imply chronic illness sufferers are somehow 'undeserving' of love generally tend to stem from our own insecurities that are either deeply ingrained and/or exacerbated due to our conditions or brand new and brought to the fore by changes in our bodies due to treatment, symptoms, or even surgery. All of these elements in living with an illness are rife in changing our perception of ourselves and can serve to lessen our self-confidence on a massive scale. When you struggle to 'love' yourself in the first instance, that old adage can ring true; how can you expect anyone else to love you back? But wait, that's not *entirely* true, is it? If someone *loves* you, or at the very least wants to spend time with you, then shouldn't they help you get back the confidence you've sadly lost? Shouldn't they be able to see your best qualities even when you can't? This is more than likely the case in a loving relationship, but we as the 'sick' ones can't often see such basic kindness even when it's staring us in the face.

These feelings or being somewhat undeserving of love are often justifiable, as regardless if you are single and living with 584545 cats, or have been married for over 100 years [are you a Disney Princess?], you will still feel alone and unlovable once in a while. We all do. It's sadly inevitable, however temporarily it may last. We can all feel alone even in the most loving of arms. It's not necessarily about our partner failing in some way in their adoration towards us, but more about the way we view ourselves: when we are at our lowest ebb we often find it hard to see any beauty or worth in ourselves. One of the most common of these insecurities are in us feeling as though we have seemingly nothing to talk about other than illness; we feel our 'value' has decreased, physically and emotionally. We can't *think* about anything other than illness/ treatment/ pain/ the sweet relief of impending death, so it's often nigh on impossible to communicate much of anything else. We can't think clearly through incredible pain, a medicated fog, social anxiety; so how are we to expect anyone to be prepared to listen to our nonsensical ramblings?!

*

For some of us it doesn't even matter who is telling us the opposite; that we are the same person we were before we got sick, that we are beautiful, that we are strong, that we are not alone, that we are **loved**. It could be painted across the sky but until we feel worthy *inside*, it sadly falls on deaf ears. This in itself can be a cause of friction within relationships. When one half has to seemingly pour constant reassurance on the other it becomes a chore rather than a pleasure.

Maybe part of the problem is that not enough of us have people who take the time to remind us of all of our worth when we need it. Not that we should expect continuous adoration on a daily basis, but a little encouragement goes a long way. Pay someone a compliment. Pay *yourself* a compliment! You look great!! Encouragement and reassurance in our 'worth' despite an illness may seem like a desperate grasp for attention on a patient's part, but it's actually a simple and straightforward kindness that can often go a long way. Well if you need a little boost at this point in the book, I'm telling you all right now that you have excellent choice in books! And I love your hair! (Disclaimer: if you are bald; I love your head!) And let's be honest, whose opinion matters more than mine? That's right *no ones*. Glad we've cleared that up. Now let me buy you a margarita and take you to a special screening of Terms of Endearment; we're heading to first base!

*

So now that we're officially dating we are extraordinarily qualified to assist those remaining singletons (a.k.a 'LOSERS' am I right?!) with chronic illness who may be considering dipping their toes in the dating pool. But is it even possible to 'date' with a disease? Is it doable to engage in courtship with a condition? Or should we simply go ahead and re-home 25 cats, purchase the entire Jane Austen collection and shares in Ben & Jerry's and readily accept our lonesome future?

Well of course not!!

C'mon ladies, wake up and smell your modern day Mr Darcy! Actually he's probably a bad example; he walked out of a *lake* with just a badly fitting shirt on. If he did that today he'd be positively reeking of toad corpses and shopping trollies. Have some standards ladies! [Insert your own alterative man/woman you'd like to smell here].

But let's be serious for a moment here; it's important to remember that courtship when you are sick doesn't have to be any different for us than it is for those so-called 'normal' people. For everyone there are still a few important rules of etiquette to remember when courting your future husband/wife, *regardless* if you are in the peak of physical and mental health.

As I'm a real-life human woman who's had relationships with real-life human men, actual real-life intercourse (conversational AND sexual!!), and full and intricate knowledge of mortgage paperwork just in case it all goes wrong; I have shared my dating wisdom with you here, absolutely gratis girls!!

You're welcome. I just hope it helps some of you find love. Don't forget to invite me to the wedding! I look great in hats!

1. <u>**Be a Lady At All Times**</u>

Let's be realistic here ladies and think for a moment about our appearance. Whether we want to admit it or not, we all know deep down that no man worth his manly salt wants to be seen with a woman wearing trousers (YUK! What are you, a builder?!) Or *flat* shoes (or even worse; TRAINERS, eurrrrrgh!). Think for a minute about your outfit ladies!! If you can't get *that* right from the outset, how is Mr Right expected to fall in instant love with you?

As we all know, a woman's' body exists *solely* to be admired by our amour. But remember it's vital to remain mysterious; you don't want to have everything out on show like a butcher's window. Get your lovely legs out by all means, and maybe a little cleavage too if you're feeling bold! You are woman; he's gonna hear you roaaaaaar!

(But not too loudly of course, remember to maintain your feminine allure at all times).

When you laugh, (and you simply *must*) at his jokes, then do it with the aid of a dainty hand over the mouth, whilst delicately fondling your pearls, maybe even slip a delicate handkerchief in there for added mystique. No one needs to see your tonsils darling. Work a little on your laugh too in preparation for your hot date; more of a sweet girly giggle is preferable, we don't need to be reminded of our childhood visits to the donkey sanctuary on a first date. Repeat after me: *I am a beautiful delicate flower.*

Good, well done. Maybe you'll be the flower lucky enough to be plucked! Hard.

2. **Like What *He* Likes**

Come ON, who wants to hear your 'woman-heavy' opinions on world politics, literature, socio-economic progress and climate change?

Not your date that's for sure!

Stick to what we ladies are truly knowledgeable on; kittens, nice shoes and make-up! Wow him with your extensive knowledge of eyeliner and Louboutin's. That way you are both 'cute' AND informative! And who knows girls, maybe he'll also mentally note a few hints for those future Valentine's gifts!

wink wink!

Yes, he may well glaze over and audibly and visibly yawn when you recite your knowledge of MAC's latest eyeshadow collection, but at least he won't be intimidated by your intellect. As IF! We don't want him to run a mile at the first sign of your having a brain! Make sure your chap feels superior at all times; as we all know, no relationship should start on an equal footing, silly!

3. **Your Hump-story**

Now we should all know by now that when your paramour asks that age old question "how many men have you been with?" he doesn't *really* want the truth. He wants to know you are pure as the driven snow, yet with the sexual athleticism of the world's most flexible stripper. So what to do when faced with this poser?

Lie of course!

Start as you mean to go on! Look, it's obvious to anyone with half a brain cell that NO relationship stands any chance of surviving if both parties are truthful about your past, feelings, wants and needs. EUGH, can you *imagine*?!

Alternatively, you could of course tell him that your historical liaisons are none of his business and that your past sexual-history/or lack of is utterly irrelevant, but damn those fella's can be persistent! Naturally he'll (quite rightfully) grind you down until you admit how many men have ground *you*. So to speak...

So *lie!* – in the world of un-truths you can be as virginal as you want to be! Work out how many bedroom-buddies he'd think was 'slutty' and work your way back from there. You want him to think you are just unexperienced enough that he has the sexual upper hand at all times! Go get him girl!

4. The Bill

We've had a lovely meal. You've remembered not to laugh like a hyena on ecstasy. You've shown just enough cleavage to get his motor running. You've done *great*. But as the meal draws to a close we now come upon that age-old question that has baffled experts for millennia; do we 'go Dutch' or should the chap settle the bill for the lady *and* himself?

Well come on, do we really need to think about this one? You are a modern woman aren't you? This isn't the 1920's!

Ladies, you are strong independent women who are just as financially stable as your (play your cards right) future husband, politely cough up our half, and maybe even pay the whole bill if nothing else just to prove you are unquestionably as capable as any man!

...Ah but then remember the continuing wage-gap and lift that crisp £20 from your Nando's table and pop it straight back into your purse to spend on the tax the government place on your tampons later!

We don't need to shatter any glass ceilings just yet ladies!

5. <u>Back for Coffee?</u>

So, the date of your dreams is over, you've laughed politely at his terrible jokes (a skill you'll perfect over time) and enjoyed only a little of the delicious plate of salad he kindly bought you (I know you really wanted the steak but he doesn't need to know you are a fat pig *just yet!*)

He politely walks you home – what now?

Well that one depends on you of course. Ask yourself the following; have you prepped your carcass for intercourse? Shaved every follicle of hair from your body? Moisturised and deodorised to within an inch of your life? And most importantly, where are the cats? Have you kept them out of sight should you get him back here? WHERE DID YOU LEAVE THE LINT ROLLER?

He's not ready for all that just yet, you've managed to conceal the cat hair thus far, let's not spoil things. So my personal recommendation is to delicately accept a peck on the cheek like the lady you truly are, say your sweet goodnights and then if need be destroy yourself with a vibrator well into the early hours.

Piece of cake eh ladies?!

Post-date, in the early hours of the morning as you awake with a crucifying Lambrini hangover, you can look forward to checking your phone every 30 seconds in case your crush has sent a text, spend the next few hours peppered with anxiety and intermittent sobbing until he does, then the blatant lie that you're 'busy' whilst sitting in your dressing gown eating a pot noodle; thus commencing the inevitable dating-mind-games!

WHAT FUN!!

*

Of course, dating doesn't always run as smoothly as the above example. Maybe that's because you didn't take my advice though, LINDA. Suit yourself Linda; die alone.

But listen, I do hope my dating guide has helped inform you of the dos and don'ts of modern relationships. It was written from the heart and with love. Take it from someone who has won over the man of her dreams even *without* the aid of rope and disabling drugs; even *you* too can find your 'one'.

*

Exhausting isn't it though, this courting lark?

As you may have gathered I presented the above 'dating tips' to you with my tongue firmly in my cheek. The truth of the matter is that with chronic illness it *can* be hard to pluck up the courage to venture into new relationships. No matter what age you are or at what point in life, being diagnosed with a potentially life-long condition can be a confidence shaker. It can be hard to focus our brains on much of anything more than just getting through the day relatively unscathed; let alone even considering starting on the road to finding love. And even when we do find 'it' there just seems to be layer upon layer of additional stressors to factor into any new relationship.

Ideally, the beginning of any new liaison should be the most thrilling, pant-fluttering, swoon-fest. You should be giddy with possibility and butterfly-stomached at the mere vibration of a text message from your paramour. But for people with chronic illness that palpable excitement is often countered by crippling anxiety. We have to bear in mind the huge cloud of illness hanging over us, waiting to RUIN OUR LIVES yet again. Once we've come down from our dramatic high-horse and remembered that our life isn't a melodrama, it's important to factor into our theatrics that although illness is a huge part of us, it's just that; a *part* of us. The minute we accept it as a game-changer in any relationship we've already given in to it. I guarantee you that there is an aspect of your new lover's personality/life/past that they are just as anxious about as you may be about your failing body and what they may or may not make of it.

Everyone, EVERY BODY has their own insecurities, and just as you may be terrified about broaching what you see as a huge subject, your potential Mr/Mrs Right may have something they feel is just as intimidating to break to you.

Of course it's easy to wheel out that old clichéd favourite, 'If your illness puts them off they're not worth having anyway' – and of course that's true, but it doesn't stop it stinging like a genetically modified wasp when you are rejected due to something out with your control.

For example one tricky area is trying to establish when is best to tell your potential amour that you are sick. I of course mean 'sick' in the gravest, most perverted sense; you're disgusting in the bedroom and I'm ashamed of you. But seriously, you'll also have to decide when to tell them you have an illness. And by 'illness' I mean that in the gravest most sickening sense, what is *wrong* with you? But seriously, you'll also have to tell them you have a chronic condition, and by chronic… etc. to infinity. So when *is* best to drop the badly-behaved-body bombshell? Well naturally this depends on several different factors; upon who you are dropping said bombshell, the situation you are in, your state of mind. You'll never find that elusive 'right time' to break important news to someone. It doesn't exist and only breeds bubbling anxiety and potential panic attacks. But there are countless 'wrong times' to broach difficult subjects. For example, perhaps don't discuss the consistency of a dodgy stool as an opener over meatballs and Chianti, or bring up your mental instability during vigorous intercourse. But then again each to his own; those things may be a turn on for some of you, and like I said earlier you are disgusting and your mothers would undoubtedly be ashamed of you.

*

Beginning a new relationship alongside living with chronic illness although often testing and difficult, should still ultimately be ENJOYABLE. If the main feeling you have with your mate isn't one of happiness then illness or no illness it's not right. Don't let your condition stunt your choice of lover either; you are just as worthy of being loved by and loving a decent, kind human as any 'normal' person. Sickness and low self-esteem can allow us to forget that so it's important we remember to value our feelings and our heart and give them what and whom they deserve.

When you are sick and in love your relationship may have a chocolate box full of additional worries to factor in but it doesn't have to stop you and your beloved having a joyful life together filled with hearts, flowers, and painkillers strong enough to flatten an Ox.

*

But this book is about women, and as such, with chronic illness there are a few more 'unique' issues we as the fairer sex must contend with. In addition to the already jam-packed itinerary of symptoms our diseases bring to a relationship as it is. As you would expect, the most obvious difference between men and women being our monthly delivery from Mother Nature, also known as 'having the painters in', the 'Red Mist descends', 'Aunty Flo visiting' etc. etc. to infinity. Chronic illness and the effects of it differ drastically from woman to woman and therefore the impact our time of the month has on a condition is also interchangeable. For several women, myself included, symptoms and pain are noticeably more prominent during this time. Spending a lot more time on the toilet is a regular occurrence (particularly for those of us with inflammatory bowel disease), and the pain of cramping seems to be intensified. We don't feel at our sexiest or even most attractive at this time. We are bloated and pressure on our gut makes us uncomfortable and tired, we are bleeding and in pain and romance is the furthest thing from our mind. Depending on medication and treatments we rely on to maintain our illnesses, these can also play havoc with our cycles. As it stands, other than the usual monthly few-day-diet of hot baths, hot water bottles, pain killers, and a VAT of chocolate eclairs, there are few things to ease this additional pain. Bit of a bloody nuisance eh? IF YOU WILL PARDON THE SUBTLE PUN.

So as much as our 'special time' can put a damper on romance and the burning of loins, so can the majority of our other symptoms. On the flip side though, some women find that sex on the day before or when *in pain* can often help ease some of the tension. The theory being that the mind will be distracted from the pain the body feels. This is good, *in theory*, however for many women with chronic illness the issue is not so much in us suffering pain (most of us deal with that everyday anyway), it's often more in feeling the 'urge' and then finding the energy to act on it. Something that can sadly become a feat of almost super-human proportions.

Clearly every woman is different; we all feel and experience differently, we all treat the men and women we love differently, and our symptoms although common are wholly unique to us. But for many ladies, sex and relationships can be real stumbling blocks, and often spark worrying and stressful situations which exacerbate already serious illnesses. This in turn often intensifies already existing symptoms, causing a vicious sexy circle, which becomes increasingly difficult to penetrate.

OOH MATRON.

During bad flare-ups of our illnesses, women with chronic illness often have zero interest in sexual activity; the mere idea of anyone coming within an inch of you can be abhorrent when your insides feel like they've gone 10 rounds with Muhammed Ali (post-demise obviously). Some women have gone as far as to suggest they would need drugs (of the purely medicinal kind of course) to get 'in the mood', or that their sex drive has reached a serious pit stop due to life with constant and consistent symptoms.

But it's not just the chronic pain and our state of mind that can stall sexy-times. Our nerves can also be damaged over time due to surgeries, medications and treatment, which can cause loss of sensation to some or all parts of the body. Gas build-up from all the 'activity' of intercourse can be incredibly painful and can lead to abdominal cramping for hours or even days afterwards; a particular issue for those women with gastro issues.

Lack of interest in making sweet, sweet love is saddening enough for the individual suffering in itself, however factor into that having another person's feelings to consider; this can be a tricky time, regardless of how long a relationship has existed. Rumpy-pumpy sexy-times or no rumpy-pumpy sexy-times, relationships can suffer when our illnesses influence our mood. They can also suffer when you refer to intercourse as 'rumpy-pumpy-sexy-times' I've established.

*

As with most people, when in constant discomfort, *understandably* the last thing on our mind is our libido. This can be disheartening for our partners and particularly hard to express without hurting your beloved vagina-colleagues feelings. Guilt brought on by this lack of interest can quickly escalate and make for an even more difficult situation. As with the bedroom and beyond, communication is the key here. It's vital we are open and honest about what is causing our lack of enthusiasm or desire. Remaining silent on these matters (or any matters for that.. matter) allow space for the other person involved to fill in the conversational blanks themselves. That generally does NOT end well. We never know what another person is thinking, we often *think* we do, but we don't. So it's important we fill their gaps in knowledge; otherwise we leave someone we love perhaps fearing the worst, finding fault in their own behaviour where there is none, or even worse; thinking we have fallen for Greg from accounts, which just doesn't even bear thinking about.

Realistically we could spend the remainder of our sickly lives dwelling on how unattractive our illness makes us feel. But where would the fun in that be? I don't know about you, but I'd rather have more fun and fumbles to tell my Grandkids about when I'm on my death bed than pondering relentlessly about how gloomy my life is until it inevitably ends. And yes I'll INSIST any grandchildren I have are forced to watch as the life slowly drains from my dying face; someone has to toughen the little pussies up. Welcome to the real world kids!

The thing is, when things get hard and life gets swamped by illness, it is imperative we try to recall who we were before we let it consume us. Personally I know, and revel in the simple fact that there are people in my life who love me, and have loved me, long before I got sick and who will love me long after. I try to love *myself* enough to look after my own mind and body where I can, and make the most of what I now know may be a shorter and harder life than I'd once taken for granted. Focusing on how bad things *might* get or how I (or my love) *might* feel in a month or a years' time is ultimately redundant, pointless, and honestly, just EXHAUSTING.

Our time is truly best spent being honest with ourselves and the men/women we love about how we feel and what's happening to our bodies. However 'unattractive' it may appear (to us).

*

The simple truth is that there is no reason on earth that means having a chronic illness can't be 'sexy'. OK so the disease slowly killing us from the inside out may not *look* or *feel* particularly attractive; but 'sexy' isn't necessarily all lacy lingerie or red lipstick. It's different for everyone. It's whatever you and your partner want it to be. For me it's the amazing strength and determination I've gained in living with this disease. The opportunity it gives me to laugh at myself and to show I am so much more than my disease. Making the most of what we *have* and not focusing on what we have lost is *so* much sexier than all the anal beads and Playboy calendars in the world.

There is also a lot to be said for looking at your illness less as an affliction and more as a 'release' (stick with me here...); an opportunity to focus on what really matters to you, and what you need and want from that other person you choose to share your life and bed with. Material things fall to the side when illness overshadows everything; priorities change and time speeds up significantly, so we are much less inclined to waste it on bad relationships. We have a unique insight in how to separate the wheat from the chaff in our relationships and that often means we set our standards higher. Low self-esteem doesn't last forever, so if someone is with us knowing they can treat us badly because we will lie down and take it, well that will end badly. (For them; *not us*).

*

I've written a lot so far on the worries in talking about your condition to the man/woman/ blow-up doll you adore, but I've failed to factor in the possibility that the person you have fallen head over heels for might actual be a thoroughly decent human being. Such a person does exist! And not just in films starring Tom Hanks! Some people don't *care* that you are sick! Some people look beyond an illness and see the person you *actually are*. Isn't that wonderful?!

A lot of us, myself included, need to try to give people a little more credit where partners' acceptance of our illness is concerned. It's maybe some form of defence mechanism that we apply when avoiding the subject or down-playing our symptoms; if we don't *tell* them they can't reject us. We can't repulse them if they don't know about it!

But then by withholding vital aspects of our life we are also muzzling the possibility of another wonderful avenue of support and understanding. When we feel we are 'inflicting ourselves' on others we make things incredibly difficult for ourselves.

If our own self-esteem is so low we feel ourselves a 'problem' for a potential partner to solve, we begin a relationship that cannot possibly be a 'partnership'.

Essentially telling ourselves from the outset we are not good enough to be loved is dangerous not only for our own mental health but for the type of person we may shackle ourselves to. We will often begin a relationship waiting for it to end; waiting for the apparently inevitable messy break-up when the other person finds life with us too demanding. We decide it's too hard so quit before we even get head. Sorry, get *ahead*. Always getting those two mixed up. Again here we allow no room for someone we care for to actually prove us wrong. It's *always* scary starting any new romance; it's fraught with what-if's and uncertainty, but we have nothing to lose in opening up to someone, and everything to gain. If they hurt or attempt to humiliate us for it, it speaks volumes more about their lack of empathy and general douche-baggery.

When we are too eager to think the worst of someone, we generally seek out someone who fits the bill. That way we prove ourselves wrong and allow ourselves to put up yet another barrier to finding that real cant-live-without-someone, love. And that's just *the best*.

*

Personally, negative reactions aside I've learnt slowly but surely when someone shows a willingness to take an interest in my condition they are almost certainly worth my time. In much the same way I would politely tolerate hearing the plot of a Clint Eastwood film another 5485854 times for the man I love, someone I give up my time for should take an interest (even if it's of the faux variety) in the workings of, (or lack of as the case may be), my body.

Having a chronic illness does provide a great deal of clarity about people's character. We are very lucky in that respect. Of course from the outset we have no idea how a potential bed mate will cope with 'it'. The 'it' in this scenario being our illness of course, not the terrifying clown of the same name. It may seem churlish to expect someone to 'cope' with something so intrinsically *ours*, but there will be times when our lover must be there as not only our vagina-colleague, but as our carer. They will be called upon to hold the hair back from our heads as we vomit like it's going out of fashion, to take us to and from the hospital, to care for our shared pets/children/people we keep in the basement while we are medically incarcerated.

When you are in a relationship you unavoidably end up sharing everything; bills, chores, bodily fluids, *illness*.

When we look for a mate we must factor in what they *can* handle. We of course can't be the judge of that from the kick-off, but it only takes one hospital stay or one bout of incontrollable diarrhoea to allow a partner to show their true colours. We will quickly learn who is strong, compassionate and willing to give. Eager and prepared to adapt to our situation and think outside of their own needs. In an ideal world, any healthy relationship should entail two people who are equals in every sense of the word. But having a chronic illness is far from ideal, and it means that sometimes we need to be looked after. Sometimes we can't contribute what we want to our homes, families, lovers. Sometimes we simply can't be 'equal' in every sense of the word. Whether it's right or wrong (it's wrong), we will at times see ourselves as a burden. Our illness is regularly a burden on *ourselves*, so it's an easy trap to fall into to assume our sickly baggage will be a strain on another person too.

This frustration can destroy even the strongest of bonds.

It's vital that we talk to our partners about our feelings, and talk about *their* feelings. Don't assume because you are the sick one that they are carrying on their healthy lives skipping through fields with a Cheshire cat grin on their face.

They are most likely miserable too. That's not your fault, but it can feel like it. That's when we don't want to talk; we shut down because we feel responsible for another person's unhappiness. We are overwhelmed with guilt. But these are the moments when it couldn't be more vital to thrash things out – tell the person you love how you feel and let them vent back –there might be absolutely sod all either of you can do about the situation, but at the very least you will be sharing information and appreciating one another's feelings and points of view. Chronic illness can be isolating and make us selfish, so it's imperative we remember neither party should never feel lonely in a two-person relationship.

As human beings with insecurities and anxieties, we are all uptight about love; about falling in it, staying in it, losing it. We all have self-doubt and reservations, but the right person will stand by our side as those concerns just gradually fall away. Whether it's difficult or not, they will strip away at what you fear, and fight with you to just let go.

At least that's what my bungee-jumping instructor boyfriend said as he tried to encourage me to jump without a rope. We split shortly after as he went missing near the Grand Canyon in what the police described as 'mysterious circumstances'.

*

CHAPS!

As we all know, us women are a sweet little mystery. Who can understand our behaviour? Not me that's for sure, and I AM one!

Hahahahahaaa!

See? It's just that sort of fun and unpredictability you've come to know and love from us. Gents, we can't expect you to understand us; we are complex beings from a higher plane. We already stoop so low down to your level that we get backache and have to pretend it's caused by badly fitting bras. But I jest of course. Or do I?! (There's that cute-as-a-button randomness again!)

Want to know what a woman is thinking? Ask her! It'll probably be bunnies and fluffy kittens and tampons anyway! You wouldn't be interested!

Something to bear in mind though is that when a woman is ill she may struggle to express the extremity of it. She will say that she is "fine".

A LOT.

She isn't fine and maybe hasn't been for several days. She doesn't say she is fine because she is looking for attention or waiting for you to probe her forcefully until she breaks down and admits otherwise. She says she is fine for a million and one reasons that she probably hasn't even thought about. From the immense tedium of 'I LITERALLY CAN'T BE BOTHERED TALKING ABOUT THIS, IT IS LITERALLY ALL I THINK ABOUT, LITERALLY'; to those more deep-seated worries of 'WHAT IF HE LEAVES ME AND RUNS OFF WITH LINDA BECAUSE I'M A WALKING CORPSE?'

So don't take it to heart when we tell you we are 'fine' and you know we are anything but. We are not trying to deceive you, you sweet, sweet dumplings. These little white lies are not designed to keep things from you but merely to protect us. It's not right perhaps, but sometimes it's easier, and sometimes the easiest thing is really important when life is as tough as that steak we made you for Valentine's Day.

Just be patient with us and let us know you are there when we are ready to talk. That time might not come and that's OK too, because some days we may just need to internally wallow and then move on.

There are really no set rules to living with and loving someone with a chronic illness; but listening, understanding and just being a calming and supportive presence are pretty high on anyone's list.

If you can do all of that, ride us like SeaBiscuit on the regular AND smile politely when we cremate your 10oz steak then consider our dance-card yours for all of eternity my handsome friends!

xo

4. A BEAUTIFUL BIND

Well now, hasn't it been just *exhausting* reading about the intricacies of modern relationships with chronic illness? I know I for one could sleep for a week right now; if only I weren't so goddamn lonely!

Honestly I know this probably isn't the best place to vent but my cat is great and fluffy and cute and all but he doesn't like bear hugs or talking about books and my boyfriend has been spending a lot of his evenings with our recently widowed neighbour who seems to "need her boiler fixed" at 3am most nights! He always comes home exhausted the poor thing; I don't know how he does it! He's just so generous with his time I know I shouldn't be selfish… he's just so eager to help others; I mean he isn't even a qualified engineer! What a sweetheart.

But enough of my problems; if you consider having MR PERFECT as a partner to be a problem! Ha ha!

Anyway, all of which stressing about love and finding Mr/Ms Right, brings us neatly on to our next topic; body image alongside chronic illness.

*

The thorniest of subjects, this one, and something a huge volume of us struggle with. Put it this way, it's often hard enough looking in the mirror on a normal run of the mill Monday morning and not disliking what we see, let alone throwing a chronic illness and all its foibles into the mix.

With a relentless illness our body is constantly changing. Often so fast we can't keep up. Hey, at least give us a minute to verbally and emotionally annihilate our new body in the mirror before changing it again faster than Doctor Who regenerates!

Our bodies change through simply experiencing flare-ups or symptoms of our conditions, to escalating illness, medications, treatments and the subsequent side effects of all of the above. Of course it's important to remember that depending on our condition, a lot of what we 'see' isn't apparent to those outside of our own bodies. Much of the negative feeling we hold towards ourselves is based in our own skewed and distorted image of ourselves.

This is a hard issue to express but I think the closest I've come to explaining this outside of my own private diary, is 'feeling *diseased*'. Those moments in which internally you feel like a slowly decomposing corpse lain to rest on a rubbish dump, (you know the ones!) and it's hard to look in the mirror and see anything but.

I often refer to myself as 'diseased'.

This seems to make some people uncomfortable and I'm not quite sure why. Maybe it's because they feel pity? They give out the sympathetic head tilt even though I haven't requested it; they do this because they don't know how to react. Mainly I refer to myself in this way because it makes me laugh and laughing is fun. It's not rocket science! I also use this wording because it feels accurate. I don't want or seek out pity for a phrase I've *chosen* to use! Correction: I don't want pity AT ALL. So it can be frustrating when a phrase I've chosen to use in order to exact a LOL or put others at ease does the opposite. I suppose I probably persevere with this choice of words because I'm stubborn and don't want to change yet another aspect of how I talk about *my* illness for the sake of others' more delicate sensibilities. I conclude that whatever is easy for me is best. I don't want to exhaust and frustrate myself delving into long winded explanations of my condition, and I shouldn't have to. I don't want to confuse and upset or embarrass others either, so trying to find a happy medium is harder than you might expect.

Being somewhat flippant about something incredibly serious is my go-to as it allows me to set out my sickly-stall from the start – I'm open to talking about this and it's only a part of me.

*

There is certainly a LOT to consider in living with a disease; therefore all but zero room to squeeze in worry about how strangers may react to a certain phrase/word you choose to use to describe how *you* feel. We have far too much looking-in-the-mirror-and-assassinating-our-own-characters to do, to find time for much of anything else really. Priorities!

As we've discussed, changes in our bodies happen so often with chronic, and in particular perhaps, auto-immune diseases, that it's often hard to keep up.

Medications can change how we look physically, which in turn can alter how we view ourselves mentally. Weight loss (or gain) can happen incredibly quickly and frequently for us, and as we ALL know, there are few things more disheartening than having to smear butter on your thighs to fit into your favourite jeans or having to tie a belt around your waist 5 times just to keep them on. The perceived notion in modern society is most commonly that 'skinny' should be the idealised body shape for women.

It's not. There is no such thing as a 'perfect body'.

For starters, *whatever the hell you are comfortable with* is the ideal body shape for women. But for ladies with chronic illness 'skinny' doesn't always equal healthy. In fact in many cases of auto-immune disorders it's a sign we are flaring. Badly. We are most likely *under-weight*; not a good place to be. It's a sign we are not eating well, not digesting food properly, we are not absorbing the nutrients we should be. It's often a sign we're about to hop back on the never-ending treatment merry-go-round, where we'll enter the medication lottery, hoping against all hope of finding a winner. You'll find that most women with chronic illness do not associate 'skinny' as a positive phrase. For many of us it's a worry, more than a victory.

'Skinny' is a description I personally detest. It's a common aside thrown at us, whereby we are assumed to take it as some sort of solace for being straddled with an incurable condition; **"at least you're skinny"** or the even more infuriating **"you're lucky you're so skinny!"** This sentence is so overtly dismissive, bitter and insulting that the people who've spouted it at me over the years have no idea how close they've come to being murdered straight to death. The amount of teeth gritting and forced smiles I've had to endure when hearing this have probably caused irrevocable damage to my cheekbones.

I accept of course that many normal people (and by normal I mean 'healthy') may wish to be 'skinny' like some of us diseased chumps. They only see what's happening on the outside, so I suppose it must look like we've hit some sort of genetic jackpot being able to shed pounds faster than your Dad in a casino. These blessed healthy folks generally have little else to consider, other than eating well and exercising. Yet still, for them, THE STRUGGLE IS REAL.

Apparently.

You see its all well and good having a big LOL-fest and guffawing at our healthy cousins weeping into their Pumpkin Latte because their local supermarket doesn't stock that Kale and Carrot smoothie that they love anymore and that's the worst point of their day. But when those of us with conditions which make it hard for us to manage our own fluctuating weight see a million and one Instagram posts 'inspiring' us with 'thin-spiration', (coincidentally one of the worst phrases in the history of man-kind) it can be, well disheartening to put it mildly.

Most of us with chronic illness are focused on making sure our bodies simply 'function' as they should, in an ideal world. We know all the kale smoothies, coconut water and vats of Aloe Vera in the world won't 'cure' us, so when we are bombarded with fake ideals where 'skinny' women seem to be brought to the point of orgasm over green tea, it just seems... well, a bit off. A bit like they are *trying too hard*. I always imagine them sobbing silently into a McDonalds as soon as they've posted their latest bikini clad selfie. I'm not sure about you but I just don't buy it.

It frightens me a little that younger, more impressionable women will wish for a life of perfect abs, handbags you carry on your elbow (WHY do you do that?!) and an undoubtedly picture perfect but loveless marriage. If these fitness fanatics are happy then great, it just seems false and that's something I find abhorrent. Maybe I'm just jealous? Maybe it's just envy at their level of worry on a scale compared to mine. If all I had to sink into depression about was how shiny my abs look in my latest Instagram post I'm pretty sure I'd be throwing a party instead.

Look, all I'm saying is live a little! Eat a cake every now and then! Add some vodka to that carrot smoothie!

Mind you, I get over-excited by a multi-pack of quilted toilet roll so who am I to judge...

*

It may sound foolish to the aforementioned 'healthy' readers amongst you, (although you've probably put the book down by now...) but a lot of women with chronic illness will feel 'betrayed' by their own bodies. This can be a tricky aspect of illness to wrap our heads around. Perhaps in particular if we are one of those GOD DAMN ANGELS who don't smoke, rarely drink, and eat kale morning noon and night. (Who are these people and why do they love Instagramming beetroot smoothies so much?)

We will repeatedly ask ourselves 'why is my body doing this to me?'

These feelings of frustration and betrayal can last for years, can flare up with our own flares in condition, but are generally most prevalent when we are first diagnosed with a chronic illness. This is the stage where we question *everything*. We wonder what we have done to deserve such a lot in life and whether we are somehow responsible for it. If we're not then WHO IS? Our parents? Our upbringing? Our diet? Our doctors? We will throw our toys out of the pram so forcefully they'll give a black eye to anyone within a 15mile radius.

This is normal and natural and OK.

It's OK to be in the depths of a tantrum like this; for a while at least. It's understandable. In much the same way we process grief; in stages; we'll go through many ups and a lorry-load of downs before reaching some form of acceptance that our body/life is most likely changing for good. Much as it can feel like it, our bodies are not our enemy. Ideally we shouldn't have to 'fight' our own body but in many cases with chronic illness we do. Often we are physically unable to exercise because we literally have less than zero energy. Often we can't bring ourselves to even attempt such a thing because our mind is exhausted and filled up to the brim with anxiety and the bluest of moods. Watching our bodies change day by day is challenging and upsetting to put it mildly and this can be compounded by the extra effort we have to put in to look after ourselves in the most basic sense. When we are at our lowest ebb we can be so utterly fatigued that the effort to do anything more than lie face down in a pillow is all but insurmountable.

Many women I chat to in similar predicaments will tell me that they occasionally 'make deals' with their bodies. I do it too and I'm probably not even aware of it half the time. When I mention this 'deal making' I refer to perhaps gentle prayer, and those promises we make internally that we know we are very unlikely to have the ability to keep. I've 'promised' my carcass so many things over the years I'll still be repaying its debt long after I've shifted off this mortal coil and descended into Hell.

I've 'promised' my body: I'll eat better, I'll exercise more, I'll never eat again, I'll eat more, I'll swim/dance/bang more. I'll DO ANYTHING YOU WANT if you just let me have one day without pain, one day without immobility or nausea.

One blessed day without a symptom.

I have had those days, albeit they have been few and far between, but I know deep down it's solely down to luck rather than any prayer or gentle persuasion. This knowledge doesn't stop the silent pleas, the weepy promises made in vain. It's maybe because we often treat our condition as an outside body, outside of our... body. It's easier to have *something* to blame; *someone* to beg for mercy.

Whatever the reason, the bottom line is that whatever beings you comfort is what you should do. That's different for all of us and shouldn't be up for judgement. We're all just trying to make it through, in our own way.

*

As well all know, feeling good in your own skin is hard to do for most of us, add into the mix a chronic illness that we can't control and it's a recipe for a confidence-crushing, never-rising soufflé. Maybe it's Maybelline, maybe it's a crushing self-esteem demise brought on by a crippling illness. Who can tell?

Any form of life-changing illness is a hard thing to come to terms with, but the idea of it being incurable is often a detail that is nigh on impossible to accept. I suppose that's not entirely a bad thing; it allows us to maintain a semblance of hope that one day there will be a cure for whatever condition we live with.

In most cases that is all it will be; hope, but there is very little wrong with having a sprinkle of it to carry us on our merry way. Especially when we live in a world often so completely void of it.

Having no explanation for an illness is tough. As humans we have an intrinsic need for reasoning behind everything in order to process information. That's why heartbreak is so crucifying for most of us; if we are discarded by the person we love with little to no explanation, we are left with nothing else to do but torture ourselves in the search for one. This is often a fruitless act which prolongs the pain more than is entirely necessary (or healthy). It also takes our Facebook stalking to dangerous levels.

So using this lovelorn logic in my sickly example you see how hard it can be when the heartbreaker in question is our own body and we still have to live with it day in day out, searching for an answer we'll never get. Our body wakes up to 100000 missed calls every day and consistently replies with *"new phone, who's this?"*

Along similar lines, when we put on weight brought on by eating too many pies the explanation is clear, the solution even clearer; put down the pies and get to a gym quick-smart. But when the control of our body is taken out of our hands it's incredibly frustrating, not to mention a real self-esteem shaker.

We are often told as women we should appreciate our bodies as they are the only ones we'll get. This is true; to a point. These bodies are indeed the only ones we are given, but that doesn't stop illness and disease changing them beyond all belief. It's like dating Jon Hamm then walking in one day to find him replaced by John Merrick.

It's much easier said than done to love your body unconditionally. Especially when it's not the body we've come to know or is missing some vital parts we once had.

*

There is no one-fits-all approach to achieving a positive body image with chronic illness (or even without). In my own humble opinion, *strength* is what is beautiful. It's something often unattainable for us sickly ladies, but something I certainly aspire to. Not just of the physical variety, (although I prefer when I feel physically stronger); I want my body to be ready to battle whatever is ahead. But mental strength is vital, learning coping methods to allow us to surf over the bad stuff when it rolls over us like a massive wave.

A lot is often said of living with a disease as a 'fight'. We are all 'survivors' and our scars are 'battle wounds'. As mentioned earlier that's a great positive attitude to have, and it can make people feel empowered by their weary bodies, which is fantastic. The only issue for me with such an outlook is again in the 'fighting'. With an incurable illness when does the battle end? We will always be fighting something which has no cure, and to me that just sounds EXHAUSTING. Let's face it, we're already shattered, let's just have a wee sit down and appreciate what we have. Anyone fancy a cuppa? It seems to me that I'm consistently setting myself up to fail when I set out to 'fight'. I don't want to constantly feel I'm on the losing team. I want to work with my body to get to where we both want to be. Look after one another, and treat what I've been given with respect and care. My body is saddled with this illness and it happens to be attached to me; why fight the very thing doing all it can to keep me alive?

Essentially though, whether you see your illness as a 'battle' and your body as the enemy or not doesn't really matter. It's up to you how you look at your condition. But let's try to ensure that as women with chronic illness we tend to value other aspects of our bodies rather than solely its appearance. Relish the contentment we feel when it works as it should. Those days when it doesn't ache and/or expel fluids from any available orifice! Or when it simply takes us from A to B, without incident!

Thanks carcass! We love and appreciate you xo

*

Let's face it, illness or no illness, as women there is, and always has been, an expectation for us to 'look' a certain way. Throughout recent history, fashion and the media has generally dictated how a woman's body should appear. For those of us who are keen to keep up to date with the latest trends in clothing, fashion is a big business. Others, like me, who dress like a librarian from the 1940's, don't tend to take a massive interest in the fashion of the moment. But for women throughout history what we wear has long determined how our body appears to the wider world, and in turn how we view ourselves. So let's hop in the TARDIS for a moment and take a brief whistle-top tour of women through the ages...

1920's – Here the 'flapper' look was in. Monumental curves were no longer desired and the look of the time to aspire to was slim and flat chested; ladies wore dresses with short, shimmying hem-lines. Bit of a bummer here if our Lord and Saviour Jesus Christ granted you a Dolly Parton-esque rack.

1930's – Curves began to make a noticeable comeback in the thirties, and the movie screen-sirens to be adored were now 'blond bombshells' with shapely curves, corseted waists and smouldering eyes.

1940's – Perhaps in part due to WW2, the look of this decade became broad, boxy and was considered to be stern and perhaps even aggressive. A taller, long-limbed, and squarer silhouette was the favoured look.

1950's – Enter the 'hourglass' figure and Jessica Rabbit style proportions were adored; curves were lusted after as a soft voluptuousness was favoured over the harsher look of the forties. Large chests and tiny-waists were the body women (and probably more noticeably, men) hankered after.

1960's – Sorry Jessica Rabbit, you're out and *thin* is in. Models like Twiggy and Jean Shrimpton in the UK were quickly and fervently adored. The slim androgynous look they embraced seemed to bring with it a feeling of youth and fun back to fashion.

1970's – Now this was a bit of a party decade (and one of my personal FAVOURITES). Bellbottoms! Disco! SEQUINS! Body shape here was still favoured as slim and even athletic; one had to be to fit into those figure hugging jumpsuits when hitting the local discotheque.

1980's – This was the dawn of the Supermodel. And the decade I was born; coincidence? I think not. Amazonian, skyscraper-tall beauties stamped themselves all over fashion-show runways worldwide and immediately became the new feminine ideal, instantaneously dominating pop culture and advertising.

1990's – Those Amazonian supermodels seemed to shrink overnight and suddenly the 'waif' look was rapidly idealised. Petite and almost painfully thin was everywhere, and perhaps most disturbingly, the advent of 'heroin chic'. Bring back Jessica Rabbit all is forgiven…

Bringing us up to date, and how do we look now? Probably a mismatch of every decade that's gone before I'd determine. Attitudes have changed over the years in terms of how appearance affects a woman's status in society, but no massive strides have been taken there by any stretch of the imagination.

But bringing this fashion foray back round to living with an illness; clothes are certainly a convenient cloak to hide our insecurities behind. I certainly noticed a change in how I dressed post-diagnosis. I covered up more, I wore loose fitting baggy outfits; I didn't feel good inside or out and my lack of interest in how I dressed was an accidental reflection of that. Now I try to make more of an effort when I'm feeling good to *look* it too. It boosts my confidence and reminds me of my life pre-sickness. Dressing the way I want to and having fun with it allows me to portray other aspects of my personality than simply 'patient'. Clothes can help me feel fun, flighty, and sexy.

They allow me to show what I choose to; they allow me to exact a level of control over my body I don't often have.

In conclusion then it's relatively easy to see how difficult it may be for a woman to keep up with what's 'in'. I barely recall if I've managed to put a bra on before leaving the house most mornings, let alone have the enthusiasm to keep up to date with what shoes Victoria Beckham may or may not be wearing at any given moment. (99.9% sure I couldn't walk in them anyway).

Trends in fashion change more regularly than celebrities change their spouses, so it's borderline impossible to keep 'on trend'. (In particular if you don't happen to earn a supermodel salary).

But really why would you *want* to wear what everyone else is wearing? Look like everyone else? The body you have is the one you should surely work with, and often fashion doesn't go hand in hand with your frame. Tough titty I say, 'fashion' doesn't do one-look-fits-all. Find your own look and OWN IT as Tyra Banks might say. After all why is 'being yourself' so openly frowned upon? Aren't we all constantly fed the lines that the very things that make us so uniquely 'you' are the things to be nurtured? It's difficult to express what makes you 'you' of course when you are surrounded by TV/magazines/newspapers/adverts telling you that you aren't quite beautiful/skinny/*good* enough.

*

Thank-fully as I've mentioned, things have moved on since the unrealistic beauty expectations pressed on women back in early 1900s, but even today the expectancy on women and young girls to portray a certain image is apparent and oft overwhelming.

Every image we see in the media is of the 'favoured' [by whom I'm not entirely sure] look – slim yet curvaceous, long glossy hair, next-level beautiful, perfect skin, confident, perfect make-up, clothes to die for. All the while we deny the innate knowledge that pretty much every image we see is photo-shopped and filtered to within inch of its life. The models are wearing clothes they don't own in destinations they don't live with a camera zooming in on their every insecurity.

Now myself, (despite this constant barrage from every potential outlet on what I should look like), am quite happy with my appearance. *Most of the time.* Mind you, that opinion is as changeable as Scottish weather. There are still those moments when I look in the mirror and hate every aspect of what I see staring back at me.

It's important to feel attractive.

Not purely for vanity, but simply for ourselves; for our own self-esteem to blossom. When we are lacking in some of that elusive self-confidence, our view of or own appearance is sadly skewed. However confident about our own bodies we may feel all it takes is for a bad day, a nasty comment, a bad run of health problems and we're back in self-esteem poverty. We may dress up, look and feel great for around 30 seconds, but inevitably the longer we stare at ourselves the quicker we'll be bombarded with a rapid-fire series of hard 'truths'.

Let me quickly run through just a few of those thoughts to give you an idea of what it's often like for a woman looking at herself in the mirror in a pretty dress;

- Jesus H CHRIST would you look at the way that hangs on your hips! One hip is higher than the other!!

- Your whole body is squint; how is that even possible, are you human?!

- When *did* your hips get that weird shape anyway? W.T.F

- Your stomach is sticking out again. GREAT.

- Is that bloat or *actual* fat? You are a *PIG*.

- This dress is hanging on you all wrong. You look like a hotdog with tits.

- MUFFIN-TOP ALERT.

- Your boobs are lop-sided mate.

- Oh god, four boobs *and* back fat.

- Your legs are too skinny for those shoes you'll topple over. BTW watch those chicken legs don't get you kidnapped by Colonel Sanders.

- Too much cleavage on show, folk will think you're loose.

- LOOK at your daft face. Why can't you smile like a normal person?

- ARE YOU INSANE TO EVEN CONSIDER GOING ON *IN PUBLIC* LIKE THIS?

- Look, just get that dress off immediately. Stop messing about. In fact, BURN IT. CHUCK YOURSELF ON THE FIRE WHEN YOU'RE AT IT.

So there you have it. GIRL POWER!!

Fun eh? There's just a snippet of just some of the nastiness that flies around my own head mere seconds after I've considered myself even vaguely attractive. I instantly feel despondent and resign myself to wearing a bin bag with a bit of rope tied around the middle instead of ever so much as considering shoe-horning my unsightly carcass into a dress again. Actually sod it I'll just tie the rope round my neck and be done with it. I'm already in a bin bag so my gargantuan body would be relatively easy to dispose of.

Of course I jest (kind of… are bin bags 'in' yet?).

It goes without saying that a slanted image of our bodies doesn't always stem from a diagnosis of chronic illness. It can be caused by painful or flat out embarrassing experiences in our youth, rapid or confusing changes in our bodies, unhappy relationships, or simply going to a wedding and finding another woman wearing the SAME DRESS. Who would have guessed the bride would be offended at me rocking up to her nuptials in a vintage wedding dress?

Just no pleasing some people I guess.

*

As young women, we all grow and 'develop' at our own pace. There is no schedule our bodies follow, other than the vague order of things we are taught in sex-education, and we don't wake up one morning with hair and breasts and all the rest. Of course that simple fact that girls grow at different speeds is difficult enough to contend with as it is; this leaves the late-developers amongst us rife targets for bullying. We become overly preoccupied with growing up, or growing 'out' as the case may be.

For me, as a self-confessed late-developer, I was fixated, for a time, on the idea that gaining a set of breasts would make everything perfect. Boys would suddenly like me, and the 'cool' girls would respect me. For after all, what woman *doesn't* want to be respected and admired SOLELY for two pieces of flesh on the front of her chest?! A teenage mind doesn't think that logically though, sadly.

Depressingly, both of those former wishes came true; post-boobs, boys suddenly looked at me in a different way; I wasn't just the funny tomboy, I was suddenly a girl who boys wanted to take behind the bike sheds and do 'stuff' with. The thrill! But rather than being elated about this bust-induced turn of events, I was dismayed. It was a jolt from the blue; why had I been so entirely fixated on impressing people who up to now my personality alone hadn't been enough for? It allowed me the insight from an early age on how appearance can so hastily change opinion, often harshly, and it stood me (and my blossoming bust) in good stead for the rest of our life together. Rather than respect people who valued my chest above my brain, I treated them with nothing but distain.

*

Now, as we all know appearance and what we find attractive in one another is completely subjective. Some of us have a 'type' and favour certain aspects of a person's appearance over another. What causes those attractions is for a scientist from Laboratoire Garnier or somewhere equally as high-brow to explain; you don't want that sort of stuff coming from someone as underqualified as myself.

For us to deny an attraction to another person based solely on the physical is to lie. It all depends on how long that may last of course. Generally, if you base a relationship on how another person looks, there really is very little room for progression beyond one date/the bedroom. It's shallow and superficial and sorely limiting. At the root of it though, nobody is 'perfect'; we all say hurtful

things about one another. But no BODY is perfect either: why should we strive for 'perfection' when everyone has an individual idea of what that is? How maddening!
I don't want a perfect body because I haven't got the first clue what that might entail.

I just want to be healthy and I just want to be *happy*.

If that means I eat a cake or 5 then who the hell cares? Due to the nature of my condition I can't often eat and enjoy food as I'd like as I'm generally in excruciating pain, vomiting or passing everything but my colon into the bathroom porcelain. So when I have the opportunity to get pleasure from food, I grab it like the online trolls who spew bile at women's appearances undoubtedly grab their penises when Pamela Anderson runs across the beach in Baywatch. (Or whatever kind of woman they consider to be 'perfect'). Essentially I don't know what 'perfect' means, and neither do they because I'd wager the only breast they've encountered in life is their mothers and/or a fried chicken one.

But I digress. My point remains; women, and humans in general, are individuals and we all find beauty in different things. Isn't that amazing? Imagine everyone liking the same thing? How *BORING*. I'm not saying I'm personally 100% comfortable with my own body, I'm certainly not, but my post-mirror reflection has taught me that it doesn't really matter. I don't have to destroy my own confidence; there are always people out there, online and in person, more than willing to help out with that one! Thanks NaziBob25!

*

Loving our own bodies despite what strangers/ doctors/ anyone else with a pulse may say, is a vital starting place for adapting to any form of illness, and really any form of *life*. For a woman living with chronic illness, appreciating our own appearance often means we may have to work a little bit harder to look our 'best'.

Or maybe it's more about finding our new 'best'. Maybe it's about accepting our bodies for what they are and what they have become, and making the most of them. When you are ill 99.9% of the time, often the last thing you want to do is paint your face like Coco the Clown or crowbar your carcass into a ball-gown. Particularly when you are more focused on whether or not that noise is coming from your failing boiler or Death tapping his scythe at the door.

My main message to you ladies is this:

- It doesn't matter what you look like to the people who love you. I *guarantee* that.
- When your appearance matters to you, and it will, talk it through with someone who has your confidence; they might not reassure you that you do indeed look like Kate Moss, but they may well help you see that maybe the importance you are placing on it is unfounded.
- Embrace your illness, don't hide yourself away. You have *nothing* to be ashamed of.
- Try to remember that just because certain illnesses can leave you *feeling* ugly, it does not in any way mean its visible on the outside. Try to look at yourself clearly and don't get the mirror clouded by your own insecurities.
- Be proactive in becoming healthier – look at what you can do to help yourself build your self-assurance; light exercise, change of diet, box-set marathon of The Walking Dead. Turns out engrossing yourself in zombies does wonders for our self-esteem. [I can't look THAT bad *can I?*]

- Hone your knowledge of your condition; the more you know the more informed you feel, and more prepared for any potential changes in your body. Knowledge is power and that confidence and self-possession shines through whether it feels that way internally or not.
- Be open, honest, and never *ever* ashamed of your own body. It's kept you alive thus far, have a little faith in your own casing as it has done in you.

CHAPS!

You're so vain; I bet you think this section's about you, don't you? Don't you?!

You'd be right fellas!

As we all know, vanity is universal. You may think us ladies are the prime mirror-hogger's all over the land, but deep down your insecurities are just as evident as ours! If not more so! We ALL hate bits of our bodies and we ALL stare in the mirror as though it were a black hole through which all our confidence seeps out.

But hey, let's not get maudlin here; let me reassure you delicate flowers that you all look so lovely guyz!

So handsome! So manly! So virile!

Listen, it's no big deal that you haven't been able to sexually satisfy a woman since 1983 or that you've been shooting more blanks than a toy gun; you **look** great and that's our only concern! As we all know, physical appearance hides a multitude of personality sins.

If you look like Jon Hamm on the outside it gives you are rare chance to woo a woman based on your looks alone! Just imagine it! You have an opportunity to get within sniffing distance of an attractive woman; just don't blow it once you open your mouth! Said the actress to the bishop!!

Appearance is important. Therefore it's imperative you don't judge our lingering glance in the mirror as vanity. It's maybe insecurity. Just like it is for you! It's maybe us giving ourselves an internal pep-talk to remind us we are more than our failing bodies. Maybe we are taking that selfie because we feel and look great, and want to remember that feeling when we are in a hospital bed waiting for the grim reaper to pull back the curtain to our ward.

So don't judge us too harshly, and try to tolerate our insecurities with patience and dignity as we do yours bbz.

And yes your arms do look SO muscly in that t-shirt, have you been working out? xo

5. ONE SICK PONY

I don't like being thought of as predictable. Few people do I imagine. Most of us generally prefer to be associated with words like 'spontaneous' and 'impulsive'. We like to be considered to brandish an air of mystery, like a 1920's film starlet, or that slightly alluring and confusing feeling of trying to work out the scent of a Magic Tree in a strangers' car.

So when I take medication and I start to play-act all the symptoms it says in the booklet I'll have against my will; it's disappointing to say the least. I read the little pamphlet that comes with my medication mostly for a giggle. I like reading aloud the various symptoms I may well encounter, mentally crossing them off and inevitably getting round to "death" in the small print. It's funny (albeit in a fairly dark way I grant you). But a dark sense of humour tends to fit well in living with a chronic illness.

It's a sad fact of life that every time we pump our bodies full of drugs death is inevitably a risk we openly, and somewhat willingly, take. Not that we think of this every time we have treatment of course, that would be incredibly counter-productive, not to mention TERRIFYING. But you see there's a delicate balance to be found in weighing up risking your symptoms worsening and/or Death, against potentially *Feeling Better*. That holiest of Grails for a chronic illness patient. For some, 'feeling better' is rarer than a sighting of the Loch Ness Monster, or an internet page without a Kim Kardashian selfie.

Therefore it stands to reason that one of the most frustrating, and difficult things to comprehend in living with chronic illness, is the knowledge that essentially we won't *'get better'*.

OK, so that's not *entirely* true; dependent on your illness you may have the ability to go into a form of remission whereby your symptoms are minimised or appear to have ceased entirely – this is generally temporary, but for some people they consider themselves to be in a state of permanent remission. This has been seen to last for anything from several months to years.

Of course what patients and doctors consider 'remission' to be may be two very different things.

No sign of an active 'disease' or current symptoms may encourage a medical professional to gleefully cry 'remission' but many patients still experience many ongoing differing symptoms regardless, meaning they certainly don't feel the benefit of said remission. Certainly where Crohn's Disease (my main illness du jour) is concerned I know many people who consider themselves in 'remission'. It's not something I have experienced personally, but the mere idea that there are some people out there with the same illness living symptom-free, gives me *hope*. Maybe a little sniff of envy too if I'm honest, but we won't talk anymore on that as I was raised catholic and don't want to be struck down before I finish this book at the very least.

Everyone goes through peaks and troughs with illness of course, some bad spells are sizeably worse than others, but as the moniker goes, incurable illnesses are just that; incurable. Therefore we'll never be 'better' in the traditional sense. We will always be *sick*, just to varying degrees. This in itself is a prospect often incredibly difficult for us as patients to begin to adapt to.

So how are you supposed to accept the idea that your life will feature sickness to some extent for its entirety?

Sometimes I forget I am ill. Those moments are GREAT because I'm 'in' them and am not thinking about/feeling/being sick.

It's afterwards that's the problem, when you catch yourself and remember that you *ARE* still ill. It's a strange feeling of almost guilt, and maybe disappointment in yourself; why are you trying to pretend this isn't happening? It IS. You're sick, DEAL WITH IT. Stop trying to pretend otherwise, it'll only end in tears.

It feels almost like you're cheating on the worse partner you've ever had.

Of course with this infidelity brings the inevitable aftermath, and if we follow on using this particular analogy, this 'aftermath' comes in waves of sadness, realisation and devastation. Yes, that may sound dramatic, but when you are 'well' and experience everything that comes with it (i.e. some semblance of NORMALITY) it can be a crushing blow to go back to your rea-*ill* life.

I'm pretty sure chronically ill people, or at least 99.9% of them will know exactly what I'm talking about. If you don't that's ok too, it's no deal breaker!*

*JK you're dead to me

But this issue, and it IS an issue, is one that can set off another discouraging loop of negative feelings. It's hard enough at the best of times to see the bright side in living with chronic illness without the feeling that you are forced to start from scratch every time you have a singularly positive experience. This feeds into a thought process I'm certainly guilty of too; which is the "I'll pay for this later" stance.

Allow me to explain.

Let's say we are out to dinner, we're enjoying the food; it's delicious and we'll even have a drink or two! *(I KNOW!)*

But then we remember; we have useless bodies that will expel this food and drink at a rate of noughts in a mere matter of hours. We will feel distinctly AWFUL in the morning, like the World's Worst Hangover Champion. We'll be bloated and our dress will look ridiculous. We will be EXHAUSTED for days.

Have I ruined your appetite yet?

It's not easy with all that foreknowledge of what's to come to simply bat these thoughts away and enjoy living in the moment. Live! Laugh! Love! INEVITABLY DIE. You get the general idea. This outlook can make itself known in all manner of activities; work, sport, hobbies, sex. It's a hard one to snap out of. The idea that even genuine moments of joy can be tainted by the anxiety of what's to come is disheartening to say the least. It's something most people don't have to consider.

With chronic illness we have to be careful so often with what we eat/drink/do, that it can ruin an evening before it's even begun. Hey *'Only if you let it!'* I hear you cry, and you are partially right of course; but not letting anxiety take-over is MUCH easier said than done.

*

So let's touch upon this in a bit more detail.

Anxiety can be a major issue in living with a chronic illness. Really it can stem from any of the topics we've covered in this book so far or simply from the oft seemingly insurmountable pressure of living with an illness day to day. Using my own unpredictable insides an example, my own issues with anxiety can be caused, or at least exacerbated by the intimate nature of 'where' my main symptoms come from. Obviously its well-known bowels are not exactly a hot topic of conversation unless you're a Gastroenterologist, suffer from Inflammatory Bowel Disease, or /and are me.

Most of us want to keep the more gruesome details of what goes on behind closed (bathroom) doors exactly that. There's nothing wrong with that of course – choosing to be open about your condition is no more 'shameful' than keeping quiet about it. I'd never preach to anyone that they *should* shout from the rooftops about their illness – I generally just encourage people to be open with the people they love so they can build a support network who 'gets it'. If you choose to talk with the wider world about what you experience then great – not everyone can, or wants to and that's entirely their right.

But silence about your suffering often intensifies anxious feelings.

With a bowel condition for example, anxiety comes in floods (pardon the pun) – where is the toilet when we're in a new place? What will be on the menu when we go to a restaurant? How long do we have to be here when we already don't feel comfortable? Will my dress hold up when I start to bloat like a beached whale? *Is it noticeable that I feel like death?* I've personally always been quite an anxious and nervy person generally, but since my illness took hold, that increased ten-fold. I've also become a sub-par rapper it would seem.

This all doesn't necessarily mean everyone with a chronic illness will become a jabbering anxious mess like me, but it's something to bear in mind if you *are* feeling unlike 'you' every so often. Anxiety manifests itself in many ways, from the mild; sweaty palms, nervous glances, discomfort in normal social situations, to the extreme; feeling physically sick, abject paranoia, leading to or aggravating depression. When you start to feel anxious it can make the simplest of tasks seem nigh on impossible. Making phone calls for example: it's not 'normal' to break into a sweat when your phone rings, but it *is* when you suffer from anxiety. You'll put off menial tasks because they suddenly seem MAMMOTH. They're not, but they'll *feel* it, and that's where the difficulty is; trying to reconcile the simplicity of an activity with your state of mind causing it to seem utterly overwhelming.

You'll *know* that when you do successfully conquer one of these scary tasks you'll feel so great, but that doesn't make it any easier to actually get round to it in the first place. You can find yourself in a vicious cycle of beating yourself up for your inability to perform the most straightforward of tasks without sweating like a dog in a ball shop. Things you 'should' be able to do often become challenging and that's ok, just accepting that fact is often enough. Asking for help or just trying to find ways to calm and focus your brain are a great place to start instead of mentally reprimanding yourself for being incapable.

Anxiety and chronic illness go sweaty palm in sweaty palm.

It's hard to tell where one ends and the other begins, much like the Human Caterpillar. Although as it is such a common 'modern' complaint, like most 'invisible' illnesses it can still be incredibly misunderstood, dismissed as trivial and even discounted entirely. It's easy to understand why having something you are struggling with brushed off as invalid or unimportant can be a real problem. Anyone having the courage to speak on how they are struggling is only able to do so knowing there is support waiting at the other end. When that safety net is removed we are left in a silent, panicked limbo.

But yes I hear you, all of this is well and good but what use am I to you if I can't offer you some advice? Well finding the cause of your anxiety is a good place to start of course, as with most mental health issues, but if it's something you can't eliminate (like a *chronic illness* for example), where to go from there?

Where anxiety is concerned, depending on the severity of it of course, there are certain coping mechanisms we can attempt to practice in order to ease the worst of it. So here are a few tried and tested tips that may work for you too.

Get Physical

Depressing as it sounds because EUGH, YUK; exercise can certainly have a positive impact on not just our physical but also our mental wellbeing. Light, non-strenuous activity is always welcome wherever possible, if for nothing more than the mood-boosting hormones it produces. Gentle exercise also helps to burn off excess adrenaline, is a great distraction, and most vitally where anxiety is concerned; helps us escape our own heads for a while. Having a distraction which focuses the mind in this way is excellent for giving yourself a chance to put things in perspective. Also the simple act of actually carrying out some activity rather than putting it off or finding excuses yet again can be a real self esteem boost.

Kind of Magic

I've spoken a little already on the simplicity of **kindness** and how *good* it feels, but it's also a smashing way to take our minds off our own concerns. Whether it's our health, work, relationships, money, WHATEVER, that may be causing our anxiety, at the root of it we're essentially over-concerned with ourselves. Doing a nice thing for another person is an effective and simple way to help us calm anxiety. Diverting attention away from ourselves and onto helping others also increases our levels of those 'feel-good' hormones we find in exercise and in petting 500 kittens. These acts of kindness don't have to be helping old ladies across the street or putting your coat over a puddle to allow your lover to cross unfettered (it's not the 1920's lads and coats are expensive!), they can be as simple as paying someone a sincere compliment or helping someone with something at work. Start small and see how it feels. Coincidentally the same approach I use with sexual partners.

Look on the Bright Side

When we are anxious it often feels as though our brains are picking out only the negatives. We ponder to extremes the potential things that can (and WILL) go wrong, the dangers, the worst possible outcomes of any situation and fail to temper any argument with a positive. This is where we can try to apply what's known as 'cognitive bias'; where we unconsciously try to find evidence to support our beliefs. For example when all we think are negative thoughts, we will consistently search our minds for clarity that we are right – 'this will happen because of this' etc. We can work to change this into a positive way of thinking by changing the things that we tell ourselves. Start small, by telling yourself that "this will work out" and try to notice the ways in which your brain will prove this to be true. Coincidentally the same approach I use with sexual partners.

Take a Break

Our minds and *especially* our bodies, are not always adapted for this fast-paced world we inhabit. Everything and everyone are going at full speed all day long. It's natural that we all need breaks and 'time-out' to function at feel at our best. Something we often forget and that is very important to remember is that both rest and activity are equally as important. Ensure that you schedule in enough time for *yourself* throughout your day; a little light exercise, some time outdoors, calling a friend, maybe evening listening to some relaxing music or some meditation if you're that way inclined. Try to treat your 'you' time with the same level of importance as your work, not as a rare luxury. Coincidentally the same approach I use with… yeah you get the general idea there.

Feeling Good

During times of anxiety our minds are a messy mass of overthinking. 'What if's' become commonplace and those aforementioned negative thoughts take pride of place at the forefront of our brain. Physical sensations that go hand in shaky hand with anxiety such as a racing heart, sweats, 'butterflies' in the tummy, etc., will often only serve to exacerbate the anxious thoughts. We tend to use thinking to escape our feelings, leading to an overactive mind and making us feel even worse. So this is where it can be useful to try and 'tune in' to our feelings. Devote some attention to how you feel emotionally, as well as any sensations in your body. Focus on tuning into them as an escape route to overthinking them. It's a far more effective course of action and helps you come to the realisation that you can indeed *handle* your feelings. The more attention you pay to how you feel you'll hopefully start to notice they change all by themselves.

Paperback Writer

Anxiety can often feel like being trapped inside your own head; held hostage by fear. Those who suffer from anxiety have a tendency to mull over the same worries over and over, much like me with my Jon Hamm scrapbook. Something that has always worked a treat for me, and for many others, is putting pen to paper and banishing your thoughts to an A4 purgatory. OK so no one is expecting you to pen the next Great American Novel, I'm merely talking a journal entry of sorts, or even a stream of consciousness where any thoughts and feelings that come up for you are scrawled out. It's amazing to establish once things are out of our heads they can begin to appear much less threatening, and allow for a clearer perspective. If you're a stationery addict like me, then it's also a great excuse to treat yourself to some beautiful new notebooks.

Present Tense

Ok so this one I've saved for last as I was reluctant to mention it at all, if for no other reason than my Dad will probably think I've joined a commune wearing a flower crown and smoking a "funny cigarette". But 'Mindfulness' is now commonly considered one of the fastest ways to calm anxiety and enjoy living 'in the moment'. A huge aspect of anxiety is the fear or unease about what could happen in the near/distant future. When we practice mindfulness and 'being present' it's like exercising a muscle; the more we do it the easier it becomes. So what is this mindfulness I speak of? Well you don't necessarily have to practise meditation to be more present (although that's also a great idea), but more just pay a little more attention to whatever you're doing. Being present is really just that; being in the moment and taking the time to acknowledge it fully. Focus on the 'experience' of an activity; the sights, smells, the taste, colours, textures etc. I like to practice this technique when I'm eating a chocolate éclair, it generally doesn't have any effect the first 5 though, and it's usually on my 6th eclair when I really feel it kicks in. If you're really focused on what you're experiencing it has the effect of calming the mind down and stopping you from worrying too far into the future. For example about how bloated you'll be after that 6th chocolate éclair.

*

Now as we've most likely established, it's very important for our health and wellbeing that we recognise the importance of checking in on our mental health. I do hope you've been listening Linda because this is important. Jesus, Linda. This improvement often starts with cultivating our feelings of self-worth. It stands to reason that when our self-esteem is higher, not only will we feel better about ourselves, but we also become more resilient. More prepared to 'fight' and more assured of our own abilities. If we are rejected romantically, or suffer a set-back at work for example, we are much less likely to be affected by it when our self-esteem is on top-form. These common day-to-day issues become less painful and easier to bounce back from when we value ourselves. For example when Jon Hamm files yet another restraining order against me, I take it on the chin now rather than weeping into a bucket the size of a small child.

An important point to remember while we are both her in the moment and I have your undivided attention, is that with a higher level of self-esteem we are also less vulnerable to anxiety and to the escalating mental health issues that can stem from it. We can stem the flow of mental-nastiness and self-doubt, simply by working on our own confidence first and foremost.

However, delightful as it surely must be to hold this infamous self-esteem in abundance, it would seem improving it is often no easy undertaking. Despite the endless barrage of articles, programmes and products we encounter day in day out promising to help us enhance our self-esteem, they often fall flat, and some even make matters worse. A huge part of the problem here is that our self-esteem is frequently as fragile as Bambi on ice to begin with. It can fluctuate daily, if not hourly. Our self-esteem is essentially ground in our own personal feelings about ourselves as well as how we 'view' ourselves in specific areas; in the workplace, in our friendship groups, in relationships. We place a huge onus on our own abilities and having them brought into question can be majorly smarting and cause a huge dent in our self-confidence. Not that I'm implying we should skip through life lying about our opinions of one another of course; the last thing we want is to create a globe run by narcissists...

You see having high self-esteem is of course a *good thing*, but much like alcohol, Nutella and heroin, only in moderation. Very high self-esteem, like that of those aforementioned narcissists, is often quite brittle. These people may feel great about themselves much of the time but they also tend to respond negatively to criticism and this leaves them extremely vulnerable. Nevertheless it *is* possible to improve self-esteem if we go about it in the right way. If you need it, here are a few tried and tested ways to help boost yours:

1. **Learn to graciously take (and accept) a compliment**

This doesn't sound difficult does it? But for many of us it is a painful and uncomfortable experience and one which we brush off faster than a wasp on a croissant. The issue here is that when we feel bad about ourselves we tend to be much more resistant to compliments; despite the fact that at our lowest ebb is when we most need them. My theory is that we should set ourselves a mental goal to tolerate compliments when we receive them, even if they make us feel uncomfortable (and they will). It's also important to remember that this shushing action we enact when someone compliments us can also be hurtful and insulting to the other party. One of the best ways to avoid that reflex reaction of batting away compliments is to prepare simple set responses and train ourselves to use them automatically. Possibly think along the lines of *"Thank-you!"* or *"How kind of you to say"* or *"You're bae"*. Ok maybe not the third one, I'm just trying to keep my finger on the pulse here. This acceptance becomes easier and almost second nature after time, I promise. Over time that impulse to rebuff or deny a compliment will begin to fade and this is a nice indication your self-esteem is getting stronger. Also I love what you've done with your hair.

2. **Use 'Positive Affirmations' correctly**

On the flipside of the acceptance coin, we find 'positive affirmations'. Before you put the book down thinking I've turned new-agey and have joined a cult in the desert wearing only flowers plucked from a giant cactus and a loin cloth because "clothing restricts my freedom of expression"; all I mean by this is a little light reinforcement of your own self-worth. This idea of positive reinforcement works for some, but can become an issue when our self-esteem is very low; the idea of telling ourselves we are "the best thing since sliced bread!" can seem trite and totally contrary to our existing beliefs. Also INACCURATE because there is NOTHING better than sliced bread, don't be an idiot Linda. Positive affirmations can work when we apply them to occasions where our self-esteem perhaps lags a little. For example change *"I'm going to win!"* to *"I'm going to do my best!"* – don't set yourself up for a fall unnecessarily but don't give up entirely. Make these affirmations more believable and more about perseverance than achievement.

3. **Identify your competencies and develop them**

This works particularly well in the workplace, and it may sound too much like hard-work but then as our parents always tell us, nothing good ever comes easy. Except your boyfriend Linda, (so I've heard anyway). When we look at how self-esteem is built, a huge part of it stems from demonstrating real ability and achievement in areas of our lives that *matter* to us. For example if you pride yourself on being a good cook, throw more dinner parties. If you're a good writer, write more, let people read your writing. In short, figure out your core competencies and find opportunities and careers that accentuate them. It doesn't take a brain-surgeon to work out that doing something that you're good at, makes you feel good.

4. **Reject self-criticism and introduce self-compassion**

I can almost hear you now: 'LOL'ing your wee socks off at this suggestion. You see when our self-esteem is low we are much more likely to damage it even further by being self-critical. Since our goal is to *enhance* our self-esteem rather than pummel it into the ground where it is left to wither and die like all of your hopes and dreams, we need to substitute self-criticism with self-compassion. Self-criticism occasionally serves a purpose of course, in *very* small doses; we sometimes need to reflect on our actions and that can often be looking at them from a standpoint of constructive critique. (Note the importance of the word *constructive* there). Specifically, whenever your self-critical inner monologue kicks in, ask yourself what you would say to a loved one if they were in your situation (we tend to be much more compassionate to our friends than we are to ourselves) and then begin to direct those comments back to yourself. Doing so will avoid damaging your self-esteem further with overtly critical thoughts, and help build it up instead with a little care and self-kindness.

5. **Reaffirm your real worth**

Although we may beat ourselves up internally for every little thing we do NOT being magic, its vital we take some time every so often to remind ourselves we are good people worthy of good things. A simple way to do this is to make a list of qualities you have that are meaningful in their specific context. For example, if you got rejected by a date, list the qualities that do in fact make you a good relationship prospect, despite what your ex says, he doesn't even know how to tie a tie correctly, the loser. For example, being loyal or emotionally available; list the qualities that make you a 'catch' and you'll find they are plentiful. If you failed to get a work promotion, list qualities that make you a valuable employee (you have a strong work ethic or are responsible). If you want to elaborate on this task then choose one of the items on your list and write a few paragraphs on why this particularly quality is valuable to both you, and likely to be appreciated by other people in the future. Do the exercise every time you need a self-esteem boost. This one may seem silly and maybe even trite at first but this is for you and you alone, be honest and you'll find much more to love about yourself than perhaps you realise.

Look, my tips are there to help you but much like socks and penises, are by no means one size fits all. What works for some may not work for others. But the bottom line is that improving self-esteem requires a bit of work, as it involves developing and maintaining healthier emotional habits. But in doing that extra work, and especially by doing so correctly, I'm pretty sure you'll find it undoubtedly provides a great emotional return on your investment. I take cards, cash, PayPal or kittens.

*

I speak to you of course not as someone who is an 'expert' in living with anxiety, self-esteem or even in a wider spectrum mental health issues as a whole. I'm not really an 'expert' in anything if truth be told. Other than cats perhaps and even then there is still *so much* to learn from those little fur-balls! Cats would tell you though, if they could talk, (and I hope to GOD I'm alive when that technology is introduced) that they have an innate ability to help ease sadness. They are seasoned pros in reducing blood pressure and making people feel that giddy feeling you get when you fall in love. So my knowledge of cats makes me incredibly qualified to talk to you about depression. Grab your nearest kitten and buckle in.

Joking aside, it's something I experience first-hand on an almost daily basis; be it lulling into periods of depression myself or handling loved ones who suffer.

I'm not sure which is harder; having it happen to you, or watching someone you care for have it happen to them. Probably the latter I'd wager as you're usually distinctly lacking in treating yourself as priority number one when depressed. But living alongside an illness doesn't necessarily make you an authority on it; it merely allows a unique insight others may never have.

Great songwriters, poets and authors throughout the ages have attempted to describe how depression *'feels'*. Some of them weave fantastical (and oft accurate) images of the illness we commonly refer to as the 'black dog'. Cartoonists and illustrators try to convey how all-consuming the illness can be. Some of their words and pictures do make us *feel*; they reduce us to tears and make our hearts ache for our loved ones. They make us *feel* things deeply.

I don't often talk massively about my own struggles with depression. Mainly as for the longest time I didn't consider the feelings I have to be as intense or serious as to be referred to as 'depression'. But then you don't *have* to be 'intense' and 'serious' to feel depressed. We don't have to put ourselves in an imaginary box or give ourselves an imaginary label. We just have to find the strength to admit our own feelings to ourselves and those around us. Openly admitting 'I'm depressed' doesn't change me in any way; no more than saying I have a chronic illness does; although it doesn't always come as easily.

I wouldn't profess to possess the intelligence or wordsmithery (see, I don't even think *THAT* was a word), to attempt such a feat as to 'describe' depression. Although if I'm being honest here, that's not really the main reason why I don't feel I can describe how it feels to be depressed; it' because it's a feeling I find impossible to put my finger on.

It doesn't have a description in my eyes; it just *is*.

I suppose the closest I could come to expressing my own personal experience of depression is a feeling of being on the outside of your own body and mind. That sounds entirely more new-age-y than I intend it to, but the point remains.

For example, when I feel my blue moods loom I realise I don't feel 'at home' anywhere. I don't feel a connection to anyone or anything. I know in these moments I am loved and am capable of love but I can't *feel* it.
My emotions are unexpected. I cry out of the blue and I don't know why. I understand saying this must be incredibly sore for the people who love me but it isn't a slant on anyone. Because when I am depressed I can't feel *anything*. I assume that is the crux of it really; it's a feeling of losing yourself. Nothingness. I suppose that's not entirely true; I do feel *something* – mainly frustration and anger. I'm waiting to come through it and I don't know what *it* is. I know I've been here before but it never feels quite the same. And it always, always feels like it will never end.

Clinging to the fact that I know I have been here before, made it through the other side, that it *has* and *will* end is all I have to sustain me. Depression makes you question everything. Why am I with this lover/friend/blow-up doll when it makes me unhappy? 'When *IT* makes me unhappy' - And therein lies another hindrance of the depressed individual; finding someone or something else responsible for your unhappiness. That's generally a trap we fall into because it's often easier to have someone/thing to blame for us feeling so inexplicably awful. It's easier to accept this has been thrust upon us for a reason, than to come to terms with the fact that this is a form of mental illness. Living with a chronic illness of course allows for a veritable banquet of these 'excuses'. I understand of course that it is entirely logical that one can exacerbate the other; stress intensifies my disease and my disease intensifying brings the blue moods. It can be a vicious circle that never ends. Much like that time I tried to learn how to hula-hoop.

I suppose even today there is still very much a skewed image of mental health issues in the wider world. These people should be in dark rooms, despairing of their lot while watching the rain fall as All By Myself plays loudly in the background shouldn't they?
The truth is, depression, like my invisible illness, is concealable. Easily hidden with a smile and a laugh. An 'I'm fine!', or excuse upon excuse as to why you

are cancelling on your friends yet again. It can go unnoticed for lengthy periods – if those around you don't know what you are going through and you are unable to tell them you're often left rummaging around alone inside your own head. Not the best place to be when it's your state of mind that's the problem.

If you have someone in your life with depression the key is really in trying not to judge them. It's in not trying to assume what they must be feeling, or to 'fix' them. You can't.

Try instead to pick up on little things, those little aspects of their behaviour that may at first glance seem irritating or obtuse, but on second glance give an insight into why they are acting the way they are. For example, don't take them cancelling a night out as bailing on you *again* or as some sort of personal affront on *your* character – ask yourself if the reason they have given you smells like bullshit because it's an excuse for them to avoid human contact. If it is that's OK – and they are letting you down gently with a little white lie. This in their eyes is always preferable as there is no denying that it's easier than trying to explain over text/phone/face to face that they feel unable to get out of bed, let alone twist the night away with you.

When living with chronic illness this comes to the fore perhaps more readily, or can on the other side of the coin be more difficult to pick up on. When there are constant and day to day symptoms elsewhere, it becomes hard to pinpoint if we are just unhappy at being ill, or if we are slipping into something more sinister.

When you feel deeply unhappy it's *hard* to talk about. Sometimes you feel desperately that you *want* to tell someone how hard you are finding things but the words just cannot make their way out. But it's crucial that we **keep trying**. Don't assume that whomever you open up to won't know what to say, or that you'll make them feel awkward, or even that you will ruin a friendship. You won't.

If you are the one we are finding it hard to open up to, when you know someone you love is struggling; **persevere**. Don't give up on them. Don't give up when they snap at you, cry on your shoulder, and take things out on you. They don't mean it and deep down you know that; because you know *them*. Don't berate loved ones for not contacting you sooner – there are a million and one reasons we couldn't – most commonly it's a struggle to get out of bed let alone call a friend and weep openly down the phone. You don't have to know 'what to say' either; there are no right or wrong answers. If someone reaches out to you because they are struggling, or maybe they don't but you know they want to, please don't give into awkwardness or the trap of not knowing what to say so saying nothing. Talk to them and let them talk to you. It's essential and can be the difference between life and death.

*

CHAPS!

So you think it's just us ladies who are neurotic maniacs?!

WRONG AGAIN LADZ!

We know you are just as bad as us. If not worse! We also know you won't admit it and that's fine, we can do the 'who's-crazier-than-who tango' 'til the cows come home if you like, but it won't help us live in blissful harmony will it? So let's try and accept one another for whom and what we are shall we? Let's help one another live as partners rather than one of us having to wear the trousers. Because let's face it, we have MUCH better legs than you, in skirts or trousers.

How about for starters we stop referring to one another as 'crazy? Maybe we are acting in a way you wouldn't consider 'normal' because we are unhappy or sad or in a shit-ton of pain?

Ask us.

Don't judge us for our answer and don't assume you know how our mind works, because you truly DO NOT. But hey, no sexism here! – I don't profess to know how a gentleman's mind works either! Although I guess it mainly involves a lot of cars, boobs and punching/kicking things/other men.

Chronic illness for anyone, male or female is HARD WORK. It can be a terrible burden on mental health, in particular if you are already someone with a fragile mental state. So just be kind. It really is that simple.

Also, our eyes are UP HERE BBZ. xo

6. I'VE GOT THE (GIRL) POWER

It's hard being a sick girl in a modern world.

Therefore it's of incredible importance that as women we value one another, educate each another and help one another up instead of knocking each other down. Unlike Chumbawumba we can't always get back up again so easily.

On the whole my personal experiences of other women within the health community in particular have been extraordinarily positive. They've helped me in immeasurable ways, to feel less alone, less 'ashamed' of my condition (and my new ever-changing body), and some have even educated me in ways a doctor doesn't have the time, or perhaps inclination to. (Albeit, with much more colourful and gruesome language). We often learn more about our conditions from our fellow patients than we do from medical professionals; after all we are the one coping with it day to day. So it's important we treat one another with delicacy and care. We are all going through our own pain in our own way.

Our treatment of one another within these environments is on the whole amazing. We learn quickly what we need from one another and where to get it; how to help one another without being overbearing. I guess for clarification here I refer more specifically to health forums, meet-ups linked to your condition, online settings such as Facebook and Twitter. When you are diagnosed with a chronic illness and dip your toe into looking for help and advice you'll most likely be directed to one of these (mainly patient-led) forums. Most experiences will be positive and helpful, but you'll also learn quickly which sort of 'help' is useful and which is potentially damaging.

So most of these situations are great places to meet new fellow patients and share and learn together. But there are times when some piranhas slip through the net and can start nipping away at our already sorely lacking, self-esteem. Forums related to our conditions, social media and blogs centred on chronic illness should in theory be the most scared of places, where we feel completely safe in the knowledge that we can say anything and everything about our illnesses without fear of judgement, or for fear of being silenced and/or shamed for what 'society' perceives to be inappropriate levels of discussion around the complexities of our conditions. Much like Christian Grey smacking the shit out of our rear ends with a piece of MDF or whatever he's using these-days, nothing is out of bounds and there is no judgement in these safe spaces. We should feel free to laugh and cry and despair in company who understand.

The health community and the women who inhabit it should ideally be our own personal sickly safety net.

But within this proverbial safety net, holes can appear that can cause more issues than they are designed to resolve. Competiveness, bitterness and resentment can bleed into our 'safe-places'. Anger and frustration can spill over into these discussions and we may be made to feel small or even humiliated for our lack of knowledge or experience. We argue amongst ourselves over what we should and shouldn't say and do. We make other women feel weak because *our* symptoms are apparently worse, [yet *we* can do this that or the next thing Linda, so why can't *you*?] We shame one another when we struggle to hold everything together. We badmouth those who try to better themselves because of our own insecurities. We tell women like ME that I shouldn't buy MDF just for intercourse purposes when really you know 50 Shades of NOTHING, Linda.

So why do we often find it so hard to just share information and love one another over competing about anything and everything?

Look, as I'm sure you'll all recognise this attitude is not unique to these health-centric environments, it happens everywhere. It's perhaps just more apparent to those of us with an illness as it can make us feel that we are being shamed for not being 'sick' enough. Competitive suffering I like to call it; whereby our sickness must be ranked against that of a fellow patient in similar circumstances. Maybe you *think* you are ill but are you as ill as *me*? I VERY MUCH DOUBT IT LINDA.

Sickness or no sickness, we've all done it to some degree. Maybe not in relation to our illness, but we've all 'competed' with a fellow human, be it on the inside or otherwise. We've all felt insecure about our appearance. We've felt out of place at a party. We see what we quickly gauge to be *The Most Beautiful Girl in The Room*, and then we mentally (and most often internally) rip her to shreds. Maybe we are with another woman and we draw them into it too. Soon we have determined that this fine-looking specimen we have yet to hear breathe let alone speak is to be suitably lambasted for her outfit/hair/make-up/whatever we can find to pick on. She is utterly innocent of any crime other than having the GALL to be attractive in our eye-line. Who does this *tramp* think she is?!

Sound familiar yes? I'll bet my mortgage, cat and last PMS-induced-impulse-buy-chocolate-éclair that it does. We are *all* guilty of jealousy and insecurity, and have all acted on it to some degree. Maybe it feels ok because your victim can't hear you; but *someone* can. Maybe it's your friend. Maybe you think you've perfected it to an art where *no one* can hear you. Congratulations! But you can hear *yourself*. And it *never* sounds pretty. It sounds bitter and unpleasant. It sounds hostile and unfeeling.

But think for just one beautiful moment if we stopped doing that...

(That 'moment' isn't beautiful by the way, see if you look closely at it you'll see the make up on its face doesn't match its neck, OMG what an embarrassment...)

COUGH

I said if we *STOPPED* doing that? OK thanks.

Well for starters it would certainly eliminate the risk of hurting an abject strangers feeling's, and maybe, just maybe it would make *us* feel better. What if instead of internally fuming with envy we approached the beauty of the party and told her we liked her dress, or that her hair was pretty, and we practiced our innate ability to make someone happy just by moving our lips and letting nice thoughts drip out. It tastes so much better on the palate than venom.

Of course some of the first (and worst) experiences we have of this sort of behaviour stem from our youth. Teenagers bullying and berating their fellow adolescents in order to become 'top dog' in the school playground, or by way of impressing their peers. I'm not sure why to be honest, being a 'dog' was never thought of as something to aspire to at my school… It's easy as an adult to see these children are generally insecure and unhappy and missing something in their own lives that leads them to act out in such a damaging way, but it's far from easy when girls are at an impressionable and vulnerable age. Personally I was never a bully; I was too painfully shy to be anything other than downright mute most of the time to be honest. I found (and still find) these people abhorrent; but I did occasionally find myself drawn into the badmouthing of others. It's incredibly hard not too, no matter what age you are. However it's something that can be forgiven as a child still desperately trying to fit in, it's not big or clever but it comes from a need to impress and basic naivety. But as we age and progress into adulthood those excuses no longer fit the crime. Yes, we can of course still be anxious to impress our peers as adults, but we have learnt right from wrong, so that naivety no longer applies. As with any form of bullying it usually stems from something lacking in said bully's life. Their Mummy didn't love them enough, they feel inadequate due to lack of family finances or education, or maybe they just didn't get the Barbie they wanted at 8 and plan to burn the world down by 30. They look to distract themselves and the wider world from what they perceive they lack by pushing someone allegedly weaker or more vulnerable down. You don't need me to tell you, it's not big and it's not clever. (But I have anyway so there).

*

Chronic illness and all that goes with it can already be an incredibly isolating and lonely world to find ourselves in. Over the course of my own illness, from my initial diagnosis to today, I've gradually found the women in my life who have been unable to 'deal with' my illness, have fallen by the wayside. This happens gradually of course, and somewhat naturally. Natural wastage, if you like. I've yet to experience someone flat out screaming "YOU ARE DISGUSTING AND NEVER COME OUT FOR MARTINI'S ANYMORE SO GOODBYE FOREVER" in my face but it would certainly be more convenient and timesaving than the alternative of watching a friendship slowly decay faster than that childhood bully I have in my basement. These former friendships have slowly but determinedly ended through a gradual dry up of invites to parties, text conversations slowing down to every few weeks rather than days, or just complete and sorely sudden radio silence. We turn to our sisters, mothers, friends for guidance and support – to explain to us why we feel, look the way we do. We always have. We share through necessity but also through a need for kinship. We want to be in 'it' together – having periods, having sex, having babies, being ill. OK well not literally together, I do NOT want to witness my friends engaging in intercourse, but sharing of knowledge and experience is certainly a boon in all important aspects of 'womanhood'. Therefore if we are suddenly struck with silence and a lack of contact where there was once a steady stream, it can be painful and bewildering. If there is no explanation as to why a relationship suddenly ends it leaves our minds to run wild with theories and explanations as to what we have done wrong. Of course in 99.9% of these cases our crime is simply 'being sick'. We don't always assume someone would simply choose to vanish from our lives on those grounds alone, so we'll undoubtedly find other ways to mentally torture ourselves with what-if's before eventually coming to the disheartening conclusion that people really *can* be that shallow.

Don't get me wrong, I may sound flippant here, but losing some of these women from my intimate circle has been an incredibly painful experience. For starters the pool of women with whom I can discuss my intimate circle has decreased. But losing the friendship of these women hurts not only because I've chosen them to be my confidantes, I've laughed and cried and shared with them, but also because now they have left me feeling ashamed of something out with my control. They've left me feeling weak and useless. I'm almost positive that was never their intention, but that has been the outcome of their haste to exit our friendship. It has made me worry that I'm thought of as solely 'the sick one', and that where once I had a personality now all that remains is a prescription sheet and a diary full of medical appointments.

Is that really how I am viewed now?

It's frightening when you are left feeling you are no longer worthy of someone's time. The truth is, when you are diagnosed with a lifetimes worth of illness you *will* change. You will have a whole other barrow load of worries that someone on the outside may never understand. But a true friend should *want* to learn. As with any change in a friend's life they should make the effort to school themselves. They will treat you with compassion, love and understanding. But mainly, other than allowances for your condition, they won't treat you any differently than they did before, because diseased or not, you are still the woman they fell (platonically) in love with.

When I stop to consider what it means to be a good friend, and generally just a good human, I see strength, independence and assurance. Beauty is often irrelevant as it comes from within. Yes I know how unbearably twee that sounds but it is sadly true. Maybe it's Maybelline, or maybe you're just A NICE HUMAN BEING? How many times have you been approached in a bar by a god/goddess from on high only to find when they open their mouth their personality stinks to high heaven? It's an instant turn off and can definitely alter any form of physical attraction. Ugly thoughts make for ugly people.

Many of us enter into female friendships with the same, if not more, trepidation as we would romantic relationships. Love is all-consuming and often a close bond with a fellow female can be just as powerful. We tend to look-up to women we have a desire to befriend; we generally start from a place of respect and admiration then build from there. Those starting blocks (and/or maybe a compliment about a flattering shade of lipstick) draw us to one another like moths to a lightbulb. Unlike a physical attraction though, with female friendships it is generally our brains which bind us together. We tend to fall in platonic love with one another through mutual interests or experiences, common lifestyles, a shared sense of humour. In some cases these joyful understandings mean we are even more inclined to try to maintain these relationships, as there is no sexual attraction, but certainly an intense bond: we 'desire' one another for wholly different reasons and that can cause a friendship to often feel just as powerful as a romantic one.

From a very young age, as girls learning how to befriend our favourite playmate, right through to our teens, and on all through every phase of our lives, we will always need and yearn for female friends to share our lives with. We take care of one another; we enhance each other's lives in ways far too abundant to count. It's understandable that in all stages of life we need a support system of strong, supportive women to help us become the best versions of ourselves, help us up when we falter and remind us we are worthy of everything good in the world.

*

I tell my own friends I love them *a lot*. Because I do, but also because it just slips off the tongue; it feels so natural. There is no hidden meaning, no mind games, no insecurity, no worry that I won't hear it back and *what will that mean* and will I live forever alone with 456514251 cats. Although a close female friendship eliminates the worry and uncertainty we sometimes feel in romantic entanglements, it's generally not something we take for granted perhaps as much as we can in relationships. We get 'settled' in with a partner and can get emotionally (as well as physically) lazy. We often seem to work harder to maintain a friendship. A good friendship relies on listening, understanding and a lack of judgement. We all make bad choices in life, and a good friend should and will have the confidence to speak up when they see this happen. A good friend doesn't stand idly by and watch you throw your life down the toilet; they fetch a plunger and help you fish out what's saveable.

As with chronic illness friendship is an invaluable tool for helping keep us in the real world. All too often an all-consuming illness becomes so exhausting that we will withdraw, lash out, or simply shut down. Having someone to call when we need to vent is an outlet we *all* need, diseased or not. Someone who makes an effort to understand what we are going through is incredibly comforting and appreciated much more than 'healthy' people may ever realise. Often a friend is just a wonderful mirror into ourselves: it allows us to keep a toe dipped in the real-world and remember that we are not alone in our plight. It also stops us becoming selfish and self-absorbed. Women 'connect' with each other in a unique way.

It stands to reason then that friends are good for our health. OK so I'm not a doctor, and I wouldn't recommend cocktails with your BFF over actual medication and treatment but certainly as far as friendship goes, in moderation it's definitely beneficial to our well-being. It's pretty obvious to come to this conclusion; having someone on hand to help you deal with stresses and difficult life experiences is a weight off ones shoulders for starters. We are good at sharing; our friendly chats help us create more serotonin (also known as those 'happy hormones' that help us combat depression and works towards creating a general feeling of well-being). I no longer look at periods spent idly with a friend as a waste of time I could better spend jogging or pumping iron or some such EXHAUSTING SOUNDING RUBBISH; I look upon these 'gal-dates' as they are: GOOD FOR MY WELL BEING. I relish them because they *make me feel good*. They make me feel lighter and happier. All of that may not cure an incurable condition, but it certainly helps take the mind off it for a while if nothing else. Laughing and loving helps make us all happier so why wouldn't we want to embrace that wherever we can get our grubby paws on it?

*

Female unity and camaraderie are pure JOY.

When you find someone who 'gets you' it's like the Holiest of Grails. The same applies with a friendship kick-started through a shared illness. We suddenly don't have the same conversational barriers we perhaps have to put up when interacting with a 'healthy' friend. We can be as gory as we like and over-share to our hearts content without fear of judgement or that fated look of disgust. Or worse, the panic that flashes across their face when they 'don't know what to say'.

Women on the whole are a glorious safety net for me. They make me feel a part of something very special. The women I most admire are those who are, like myself, full of admiration for their fellow females – they pay compliments to one another, help one another when they are in trouble, protect one another from those creepy men in nightclubs, they share openly and care deeply. They don't shy away from someone because they aren't wearing the right shoes or don't 'fit in' – they relish the opportunity to learn from someone with different experiences, opinions (and shoes).

It's easy to hate being a woman though. We have the painful periods, the agonising labours, we are forced to deal with sexism, ageism and occasional ingrained hatred from men (why IS that?!). God knows I didn't like being a teenage girl much at all – especially once breasts arrived on my carcass – suddenly I was swamped with unwanted male attention quicker than Gillian Anderson at a Sci-Fi conference. It's not an easy pill to swallow when you establish that your value towards men lies in two pieces of flesh on your chest you had no say in. I worked this out from an early age – and I didn't like it ONE BIT. The men in my life (OK, boys) had previously liked me for my personality – the ones who didn't, and up until now hadn't given me a second glance, suddenly wanted to shower me with attention. Much as my teenage-girl-brain liked the idea that 'cool' boys now 'liked' me – I knew deep down it was false, a beautiful illusion – the last thing they were interested in was getting to know me – they wanted quick and easy access to my knickers and that was NOT HAPPENING. Depressing as that realization was at a young age, I'm glad I had it. It's a prime example of a good set of values instilled in me by my parents, the idea that I should never settle for any less than someone worthy of my time/vagina stood me in good stead for the future. From then on, whenever I felt I was being used for anything other than my enjoyable company and endless cat anecdotes, I knew it was time to hit the road Jack. I said LEAVE, Jack.

Of course for all it's a minefield at times being female; it not always an easy a ride for men either. The male of the species deals with many of the same issues we encounter; perhaps we just tend to talk about it more? This is incredibly healthy as far as I'm concerned; what better way to bring unspoken 'issues' into the light than through communicating them with others? Reminding young and vulnerable women that whatever they are going through is NORMAL and will get easier is vital. Talking to young girls is SO important. They are afraid of EVERYTHING and need reassurance. OK, so we all do; that bit generally never really fades, but young girls becoming women need all the care they can get. How terrifyingly easy it is to be led astray, to be flattered by a dangerous stranger, to feel singled out, be bullied, become introverted and depressed. It's so important we take the 'shame' away from every aspect of being a woman.

*

When you have a chronic illness, that shame we once felt in our youth (perhaps some of us still do) can rear its ugly head again tenfold. We can become afraid, retreat back into our shells and silence ourselves. It seems easier; to hide away, but all that does is make it even harder to gain the courage to come back out again.

With that in mind, here are some things we can all do to help women like us with (or without) chronic illness:

1. **Pay attention to what we don't say.**

So many people hide their true feelings in anger, frustration, or just over-the-top expressions of emotion ('extreme' happiness/sadness). It's important we pay attention to more than just "I'm fine!" – 99 times out of 10 that's a knee-jerk to something we don't want or have the energy to discuss. This doesn't mean you should pander to our every whim, just try to be a little more open to the other aspects of our actions.

2. **Do not bully or badger us into anything.**

A good rule for life really. Bullying behaviour generally stems from sizeable insecurities on the side of the 'bully' – take a moment to look at why you are so insistent on making us feel bad. You might not even realise you are doing it, but forceful or demanding behaviour can be overwhelming, and pressurising someone who has an additional illness to factor in, can often be a super-fast friendship ender.

3. **Remind us we are not alone**

Whatever we are going through may feel isolating but it is a shared experience and it can often help to hear that someone has come through it before us. Don't preach to us about how easy it was for you – it's not a completion here – just be realistic and honest and that will speak volumes for our self-esteem.

4. **Help us help ourselves.**

Look with or without us for practical solutions to our issues and help us to help ourselves. Seek outside help or assist us in find the support we need elsewhere. This isn't washing your hands of us; we are not superhuman and don't expect you to be either. Don't beat yourself up if sometimes a hug and a kind word isn't enough. We might need more specific help you can't give us – you can help more than you imagine just by accepting that.

*

Everyone, no matter how much front we put on for the sake of others, wants acceptance from others. We want to know we are 'living right' – that how we conduct ourselves is normal (what *IS* that?) and that we are doing everything we can to 'fit in'. Sounds just *awful* doesn't it?

Whether we are a wallflower who never wants to be noticed in any room, or the life and soul of every party; we all experience social stress. Be it nerves when attending a job interview, unease in making friends within new social circles, or anxiety over the ABJECT HORROR of public speaking. Many medical professionals will undoubtedly agree that how our brains respond to 'social stressors' can influence the body's immune system, and more importantly in ways that can negatively affect health. Certainly with conditions related to the gut this is a particular concern.

Sensitivity to 'social rejection' has been proven to cause an increase in inflammation; and although increases like this can be adaptive, 'chronic inflammation' can increase the risk of a variety of disorders, including asthma, cardiovascular disease, rheumatoid arthritis, and poor mental health amongst others. We place huge bearing on how we appear to others; often to the extent we may 'act out' or utilise a fake persona, one we think will impress those we seek to. This in itself is mentally exhausting. Chronic inflammation arising from the mere perception of social rejection is *stressful*, and it's been clear for some time how deeply stress can increase the symptoms of disease, societal stress often more than others.

Of course there are different types of stress which can lead to or exacerbate different conditions. A veritable banquet of anxiety! Generally 'social stressors' such as the death of a loved one, relationship breakdowns, or emotional/physical abuse are the biggest culprits in depression. Understandable I hear you cry! But chronic stress, such as the stress experienced daily within the workplace or a dysfunctional relationship for example, can also contribute to cardiovascular illnesses such as coronary heart disease. Who's laughing now smarty-pants?

So in conclusion, it would seem that friendship *is* good for our health!

Can't say I'm stunned at that nugget of insight myself but I'll happily accept it if it means I have another excuse to spend hours upon hours with the women I love. Knowing trusting in those women we can rely on and who will support us and care without judgement really does help us physically as well as mentally, and that in itself is vital to remember when in those blue moods when we want to shut out the world. Letting a little bit of sunshine in is always a good idea.

*

Continuing in the vein of pulling one another up instead of knocking each other down, and allowing a little friendship into our lives as some of the BEST medicine, how does this fit into our wider and sickly lives?

The problems with this blissful female love-in tend to begin when we compete and attempt to out-do one another. Of course as we've mentioned, women, and humans in general will always find our own flaws in others, and that can lead to bitterness, jealousy and general discomfort being around people, let alone other women. But it's important to surround yourself with a community of females who lift you up. Those people who make you feel worthy and leave you smiling for simply knowing them. As we've mentioned, within 'illness' circles there can be a strange feeling of this aforementioned competitive suffering, whereby we try to outdo one another with worse symptoms, scarier procedures, more horrific operations, bigger scars. There are no winners in this game, of course, sickness is sickness and finding out someone has a scar 5 inches shorter than yours really shouldn't be something to feel proud about.

There is no 'smug' in sickness.

If you want to talk about what you happen to share in common with someone else then do just that: *SHARE*. Don't compete, or mentally scroll through your medical history looking for a memory that confirms that yes, you indeed are the 'sickest'. If those feelings of competition arise in your life with chronic illness, that's fine, just use those feelings to revaluate what's important to you. Is it better to water a blossoming friendship by empathising and sharing knowledge, or to let it wither instantaneously by stomping on its very roots due to your compulsion to top the Sick List? If we are rolling on with this plant analogy I should disclaimer this by advising you all that I've even managed to kill a cactus, so thank the lord in heaven I'm better at maintaining friendship than I am at having green-fingers.

So the more we berate one another for not being 'sick' enough (whatever that means), or for not trying hard enough, the more we begin to let doubt creep in on our own abilities. As women we are already under so much pressure to maintain a home, a relationship, have a career and maybe a family, on top of managing a chronic illness, it's just nonsensical to make that even harder for your own species. You are in the same diseased boat as these other women so you have the unique ability to help someone mirroring yourself: so grasp that! Don't impress upon us that you have it worse; you don't actually know for a fact that you do – we may just be better at hiding it than you are. Maybe they can teach you some thing's that may make change your outlook and make life a little easier for you too. Have you ever thought of that Linda? No, I didn't think so.

*

I *love* the women in my life. My friends, sickly or otherwise are a beautiful, unique and exceptional pick and mix of all my favourite qualities in human beings. Women, who make me incredibly happy every day, offer me more support than a strong underwire and make me very proud to share a vagina. Well not 'share' a vagina, we all have our own vaginas obviously, we don't have a system whereby we each take turns having custody of the one vagina, I mean that would be MAYHEM!

But as we've discussed, looks aren't everything. They do not maketh the (wo)man. You don't have to look like you've been dragged through a hedge backwards to consider yourself a feminist either. Where is the rule book that tells us we are somehow unable to talk about equal rights if we enjoy wearing make-up and grooming our vaginas? Society is forever full of great ideas on what we should and shouldn't do but generally places little focus on what actually makes us happy.

So, preapproved by those sequin decked-veterans of Girl Power themselves, the Spice Girls*, here are my own Very Important Points on loving your fellow (wo)man:

(Disclaimer: *the Spice Girls are not affiliated with this drivel in anyway. Zig ah Zig Nah.)

1. **Be proud of one another when we achieve**, and even in those moments when we try but don't. The last thing we need is a continued reminder of our epic failures. We need reassurance and encouragement to get back on the proverbial horse. Or the actual horse if riding or gymnastics is your thing.

2. **Encourage one another to be the best version of ourselves**, show your friends the mirror of what *you* see in them and enjoy it when they flourish; don't see a friend doing well as a bad reflection on you. Try not to compare success, juts relish in someone you love achieving something that makes them happy and being just as happy to share that joy with you.

3. **Don't hate yourself for those times in which you feel negative feelings creeping in** towards someone you love; jealousy in particular. It can be a crushing blow when someone close to you 'beats you' to something you badly crave. Be it your dream job, a new relationship, a child. Take the time you need to come to terms with it but don't shut them out. Lives go on and friends can't (and shouldn't have to) put theirs on hold to make yours happier.

4. **As an aside of the above, jealousy can act as a powerful catalyst**. Think about *why* you are envious of someone you love; what's missing in your life that's making you resent someone so close to you. Now go and make yourself happy and don't worry about anyone is else is up to.

5. **As far as chronic illness goes, whether you are on the side of sufferer or not, try to remember to consider your friends feelings** when they are at their worst; none of it is their fault. No one is at 'fault' – it's just an unfortunate hand

we've been dealt in genetic bingo. There is no one to blame, no one to drink wine and slate for their bad perm and no one to write nasty texts to then delete them. A friend with a chronic illness doesn't want to be feel/act like this; they didn't choose the sick life the sick life chose them. They are struggling with feelings you may never understand, so don't beat them up for something they can't control.

Be patient and remember all things will pass.

*

CHAPS!

Hi again fellas! OK how to make this section about you guys... Hmm... I don't know, I mean by this point surely you've got the message that this particular tome isn't aimed at you? Nevertheless I do appreciate you sticking it out anyway, as if it were your loveless marriage.

So I suppose you hear us women bitching about one another and maybe think it juvenile and bitter. It IS. But it's also a part of human nature we often can't deny. Like most humans we fail sometimes when essentially we are always trying to be 'better'. We all say silly things through insecurity and self-doubt, just like you do when you undress.

Sometimes you accuse us of being attracted to the women we 'bitch' about. Huh! Only in your warped fantasies buddy! We are capable of finding another woman attractive without wanting to French-kiss her, you loser. Besides it's good for us to vent these feelings of jealousy at you as our partners in semi-crime - that way these negative thoughts are off our ample chests and not bottled up to explode all over Linda at the next board-meeting.

Do you really think you men are so dissimilar? Not a CHANCE matey! Men are just as bitchy as us girls, if not more so! You LOVE it. Don't deny it, we know you. I mean the amount of time you spend talking about Jim from Accounts of an evening you'd think you were in love with the dude!! Hahaha! You do talk a LOT about Jim though. It's kind of tedious. It's bordering on obsessive to be honest. Hold on, are you though?! Seriously, do not lie to me, ARE YOU IN LOVE WITH JIM FROM ACCOUNTS? xo

7. RED, RED WHINE

I always make a point of smiling politely at the gaggle of student doctors who get on the same bus I do in the morning as I make my work and they make their way to the local hospital. Mainly because I'm only too aware that one day inevitably one, if not all of them will see my anus. And if you want my advice, (and I'll assume you do as you're still here after several hundred pages), you *always* want to be on the right side of any man or woman who has unfettered access to your internal organs.

As an aside: Do we call student doctors who run in packs a 'gaggle'? Is that impolite? Maybe: "a 'medical-negligence-lawsuit-waiting-to-happen' of student doctors"? I don't know, it' just my thoughts, feel free to come up with your own.

It used to embarrass me, the idea that a strange man had seen my intimate crevices more often than my face, but my boyfriend and I went to therapy and worked through it together. Anyway, these precious anus-allies aside, it's forever important to cultivate good relationships with medical professionals where you can in living with chronic illness. It can be equally difficult and frustrating when you struggle to find that doctor who 'gets' it, but it's always an incredibly safe and reassuring feeling when you find one who does. For me, coincidentally enough it's been women who have most commonly made me feel safe, hopeful and protected following my diagnosis. It was a female surgeon who operated on me and saved my life, and it was a female consultant who fought with her peers to get me said operation in the first place. I felt powerful and optimistic with this duo of women helping to keep me alive. Not that there haven't been men who have contributed to this cause also, there have and continue to be, many! But it's these two women who have stuck in my mind and stuck with me throughout my post-surgery life.

*

It's consistently incredible to me that doctors and nurses go to work every day and save lives. SAVE LIVES. How amazing is that?! They don't worry about the future beyond ensuring that the people they care for have one. It's selfless and humbling. When I told my surgeon I was deeply in love with her and that she was the most beautiful woman I'd ever seen and also THANK-YOU for saving my life, I may have been on a great deal of morphine, but the point(s) still stand. Yes, naturally she romantically rejected me, which stung painfully of course, but she also simply batted away my grateful thanks with an "I'm just doing my job". What a woman.

Of course there are amazing women everywhere, they are all around us. They *are* us. Sometimes we just don't notice them, walking around being wonderful and doing wonderful things. These women are more than just their jobs; those jobs are just a means to and end for some or more so a vocation to others. But what interests me is what drives these women, *us*, to help and inspire people around us. It's maybe just an ingrained kindness, empathy, or learned behaviour from what we've experienced around us and what we may see happen to those we love. Whatever the reason we all do things every day that go unnoticed, often even by ourselves, that we do without thinking that mean the world to someone else. The surgeon who saved my life operated on a woman she had no knowledge of; she didn't know I love cats and eat Nutella out of the jar, that I'm the level of clumsy that genuinely slips on banana skins or that I have an unhealthy obsession with Jon Hamm. None of that matters to her, not because she is unfriendly or unwilling to learn about her patients, but because I was a job for her to carry out, a problem to be fixed. I on the other hand put my faith in a stranger because I had no other choice. We all put our faith in other women day in day out and half the time we don't even notice it.

*

When you are sick one, you become reliant on other people to help you. The future seems bleak. It's not a comfortable situation that one, to feel you must be 'looked after', particularly if you are a woman who values her independence. (Throw your hands up at me). This reliance is not necessarily in requiring assistance with mobility or cleanliness (although these things have all factored into living with my own illnesses), but more to do with keeping on track with treatment, working together to find the right treatment plan, etc. I'm a strong believer in taking an active role in your own recovery. Too many people are happy to sit back and take what is given, knowing all the while our bodies will reject or respond badly to it. It's unsurprisingly exhausting, trying and failing, it's often easier to let someone else do the leg-work. But only *you* know your own body; you live with it every day. This is why it's important to speak up. Disagree with a doctor if you disagree. You have every right to do so, the same way you would in any other human-on-human situation. They are there to help you feel the best you can be, so help *them*. Don't sit silently by as they lead you down a road you know will most likely be detrimental to your health. They are the detectives; we are the most vital witnesses. Work together! After all the body you are discussing is your own. They will close the door as you leave and move onto the next patient; you will find yourself on the other side of it still living with the same illness, carrying the same worries and anxieties.

This idea of feeling we are no longer 'in charge' our own bodies and require support is often a crushing prospect, but it needn't mean we shut ourselves off from the world. Aside from the medical and physical aspects of our conditions which can make us feel like a hindrance to those around us, a common aside of living that chronic life is 'brain fog'. Sometimes my own brain is so foggy I'm surprised it hasn't caused a 5 car pile-up.

*

This **'brain fog'** is a very frustrating and generally unspoken aspect in living with a chronic illness. It can be caused or exacerbated by the incessant symptoms of the conditions we suffer from, a lack of sleep, extreme fatigue, and very commonly the seemingly constant stream of medications we oh so gleefully fire down our gullets.

If you pay attention you'll find that this 'brain fog' can be noted in various aspects of our behaviour. For some of us it really only becomes apparent when the changes in our actions are pointed out to us by others. It can often be more easily spotted by those around us as we are too busy being dazed and confused about such things as the meaning of life and why we put our dirty underwear in the fridge again. For me this doziness shows itself in my speech; I often find my words slurred when talking, forgetting the end of my sentences, or struggling to attach the right word to the thought it belongs to. It's incredibly infuriating, and can be disconcerting in certain situations. When I'm at my lowest ebb it becomes a BIG DEAL. It becomes a major worry that I can be a young woman yet so capable of losing track of my own train of thought. I know *logically* it's all down to illness and medication, but I can't help but worry in the long term whether the damage being done to my brain is irreversible.

Am I losing my marbles already? Just how much am I aware of in terms of what is going on in my own head?

I know I forget a LOT more than I remember these days and that in itself is a frightening prospect. It's hard when faced with wading through this brain-treacle not to panic at how quickly these issues may escalate. It's just another thing to add to the Worry List and that in itself only adds to the exasperation we already feel about ourselves.

For me rather than mentally torturing myself with horrifying 'what-if's' mainly involving me in a straight-jacket surrounded by nurses, I've tried to find ways to aid my 'fog' rather than fight against it. For starters straight-jackets are incredibly unflattering and other than a pair of black slacks I'm not sure I'd have anything suitable in my wardrobe to style it out. So in an attempt to alleviate some of these worries for you dear reader, here are my tips to aid The Fog when it descends.

- If you struggle with memory loss, you can never note things down too many times. A physical reminder is vital if your brain can't hold onto information like it used to. I utilise my calendar in my phone, a pocket diary in my handbag, notes on my desk calendar, tattoos. You get the general idea; you can never make too many notes in too many places.

- For more immediate things I'll set myself reminders: this is particularly useful for providing myself with gentle nudges to take meds and/or book upcoming appointments. I set an alarm on my phone for the time I have to take medication, or for a time when I know I'll be able to make a phone call to my nurses/doctors.

- If your main concern is in possible progression of your 'fog' then keep a symptom-diary. Note down any occasions where you felt a cause for worry and detail it. List any outside factors that may have led to this particular 'episode'; changes in routine, diet, medication. This is a good way to keep a record of any escalation of symptoms and a great tool to have in your arsenal when meeting with your doctor.

Don't look on making these adaptions to your day as failure, they are designed to aid you in living as close to normal as you can. Every little helps.

*

But let's get a tad more serious here for a minute; thinking to the future when you have a chronic illness can be beyond terrifying. It can be the catalyst for a massive anxiety attack, a depressive episode, or simply another worry to add to an already overflowing pot. (I didn't ever promise I'd end on a high note…).

I've personally made a lot of bad decisions in my life; like staying in unhappy relationships for too long, doing and saying hurtful things to people I love (and people I don't), allowing myself to be manipulated by people I once considered friends, buying the smallest jar of Nutella, the list goes on. But opening up about my illness hasn't been one of these bad decisions. It's helped me educate myself, help others and learn more about my body and mind than I ever would have by staying silent. Talking and writing about my life with chronic illness has given me a rare opportunity to transform one of the worst parts of my life into one of the most meaningful and positive. It's become an outlet for me to express my fears and struggles in adapting to an incurable illness. It's also offered others in the same or a similar position; a chance to feel less alone and maybe not as terrified of their predicament, and able to face their future without as much fear. That alone makes my heart *swell* and is something I'm incredibly proud of.

So like most people I have ambitions and hopes and dreams for my own future, but at the root of my ambition is to be kind. To simply make people feel good about themselves; not to pummel other women into submission though envy, panic and my own insecurities. When that remains at the top of the list I feel less anxious about my future as I know this is one ambition I am able to achieve.

In case you feel I am showcasing myself as some sort of enlightened being here, let me reassure you that although I try to keep my thoughts of the future manageable and positive, I am too riddled from time to time with many of the same worries I know you are. I know, I appreciate it's hard to believe a celebrity of such stature as myself would be capable of the same fears as you mere members of the general public, but it's true. These have increased tenfold on the anxiety scale since incurable illness became my life-partner. Let's take a look at some of these (stop me if you've heard them before – in your own head a million and one times):

- **I won't be able to have children.** I don't even know for sure I *want* them or that the man I love does, yet it's still a foreboding concern that I'll be unable to carry a healthy child. Or simply how I'd cope having to stop my treatment throughout a pregnancy. Or worst of all; that I'd end up passing my disease on to a child.

- **I'll have more difficulty with my mobility** – yes I know that's inevitable as I age, I'm talking more immediately. I already suffer from arthritis, nerve damage, chronic pain, and this has progressed slowly since my mid-twenties, so following that rule... well I don't like to think about it for too long.

- **My symptoms will eventually become so unmanageable that I'll be unable to work** regularly and what burden that would put on my partner. Independence is very important to me and the idea of giving that up against my will is a tough pill to swallow.

- ***I'll be confined to my house*** due to ill health and slip further into depression. Another scary prospect; recovery is hard and eliminates a lot of human contact (if we let it).

- ***My medication(s) will stop working*** for me and I'll have to start from scratch or suffer the symptoms medication free. This is something I've already encountered more than once so it's a particular fear not unfounded. It's likely this will happen again in my future and that's frustrating to put it mildly.

- ***I won't be able to keep up with my partner.*** Yes there are 7 years between us and he has a *very* grey beard, yet I am the 'sick' one and I often fear he'll eventually get tired of slowing down his life to my meet my speed. I never want to be his, or anyone else's burden.

- ***I'm going to die young.*** No explanation necessary.

Fun eh?! Ok so all of those are my genuine worries and appear at different times based on several factors, including the extent of my symptoms, state of my mind, whether I've forgotten to buy the milk. They bat about my head from time to time. They are no longer constant as they once were, because I am content, in love and much more knowledgeable about my illnesses. But it just goes to show how intense the side-effects of chronic illness can be. And I'm not talking about the War & Peace style instructions listed on our prescriptions here. As we've discussed previously, worrying about anything and everything does nothing to ease or lessen the anxiety and stress of living with sickness. For many conditions it actually makes symptoms decidedly worse. So why do we do it? And more importantly, how can we look forward without fear?

It's a strange emotion. The definition of fear is as follows;

'...An unpleasant feeling of anxiety or apprehension caused by the presence or anticipation of danger'.

Fits well with living with an incurable illness I'd proffer. As I've gotten older I've realised how much of our daily lives are spent in fear.

Not to the movie-style extremes of running around screaming in a haunted house clutching whatever weapon you have to hand awaiting your inevitable death. (Although those moments *will* happen to all of us from time to time, it's unavoidable). No, I refer more to the day to day fears we all have, many that stop us doing the things we love or desire. Stop us achieving our goals and being all we can be. If I sound like a crap 'motivational speaker' here then so be it. I only want what's best for you all. I'm not afraid to say… I… I love you.

*

This fear I speak of covers all bases; from fear of the unknown to fear of similar dire situations happening to us all over again. With chronic illness there are realistically lots of things to 'fear'. The aforementioned list of my own is a clear indicator of that. The extent to which we fear these things changes based on time, experience and a variety of other factors.

I'm afraid of the future in certain ways now that I once would never have considered, but when my own sickly journey began, I feared the *unknown*- I was in agony and didn't know why. That in itself was TERRIFYING. From then on, everything was *petrifying*. Every stay in hospital, every test and procedure, every discussion with a doctor scared the proverbial out of me. Something of an inconvenience considering I was already having issues in that department.

Fear ruins lives. It stops us living.

I decided to take action when I feel fear creep in. I work on anxious feelings by breathing and 'being present'. When I get nervous in hospital I remind myself I've been through worse, that I survived it, *all of it*, and that I am here for good reason. It doesn't always make me feel joy upon joy when I'm being prodded and probed by relative strangers but it reminds me to get my priorities in order. Pain is relative and I suppose the more experience you have of it the more you understand your own tolerances. I used to be scared of needles for example, now being routinely stabbed is a part of my life so it means nothing. It's not pleasant but it's no longer a massive dread, I'm resigned to the fact that it's merely a few seconds discomfort for a good cause in the longer term.

It's important to remember that although fear is a part of life it can be incredibly damaging. It stunts our growth and spreads like wildfire amongst our family and friends. I'm not expecting any of you to deny your true feelings for the sake of others, although most married couples do it every day. I'm more suggesting we try to look at why we are so fearful and how we can resolve that. Going forward is always better than looking back, and most of our fears come from bad experiences in our past.

*

I mentioned briefly earlier that one of my own worries concerning my future is my potential inability to have children. The truth is I've never really wanted them. I *like* children, don't get me wrong, although I couldn't eat a whole one hahahahhahaa. No seriously, I only managed an arm and I was FULL! Those little blighters are filling!

Although this is a mild concern, (especially the older I get), it's not something I give a massive amount of thought to. That is until I tell another woman I probably won't have children. Then I open up a can of worms big enough to feed 50587554 magpies for a decade.

Motherhood to me is wonderful and I've adored seeing friends of mine blossom into incredible mothers in front of my eyes. Watching their children grow from squishy babies into little walking talking people has been an emotional rollercoaster. It just doesn't mean I want that for myself. And I've stopped beating myself up for that now. Stopped assuming there is something wrong with me. The older I've gotten the more apparent those feelings only stem from outsider's opinions on my womb. Of course I understand that women who have become mothers and feel such a strong pull and desire to have children can't grasp why I wouldn't want that same experience. But that doesn't make their judgement valid or my choice any less *mine*.

I know I share these same frustrations as many 'childless' women. Many are my own friends, who have the same or similar reasons as me for choosing not to have a child. The truth is other people haven't the first idea why we don't have children. I may not be able to carry a child for example, I may have experienced some trauma earlier in life, my partner may be unable to 'give' me children, I may be suffering from a condition or I may just want to lie on a beach without a toddler throwing shells in my eyes and kicking up sand. The bottom line though, my *body; my choice.* For many of these women (and men) who can't quite understand why I haven't exited a child from my nether-regions by this point, the idea that I am unable to conceive would be preferable for them. Or at the very least easier for them to understand. The idea that I don't have children because I *can't*, allows room for consideration and care and understanding, even unwelcome pity. The concept that I have purposely *chosen* to avoid motherhood is too confusing for many women to digest.

I've been told 'I'm selfish', I'm 'being unfair' to my partner, I'm 'being naïve', I'll 'realise eventually it's what I want', and I'll 'know when the time is right'. And all of this generally comes from abject strangers. It leaves me feeling I am somehow less of a woman and I should be ashamed for feeling happy that my vagina doesn't look like a poorly made taco.

(Side note: Any mothers reading this, I'm sure your vaginas are perfection)

The idea that something so obviously an individual *choice* is judged so harshly (and so regularly) is incredibly frustrating for many women without children. Even more so when you have a chronic illness which may mean you are already at a disadvantage of being able to conceive, or carry a child full-term, or worse that you may pass on your own illness to another human you've chosen to bring into the world. Many treatments for common chronic illnesses supress an already failing immune system, this requires further medication which can either be harmful to the baby or the mother or both. Starting a family for someone diseased is often not a simple choice; the factors involved can often be a case of life or death. Now tell me again how I'm being selfish.

Therefore it's frustrating when other women judge us based on their own experience. Becoming a mother isn't for everyone. It's a decision that shouldn't bae taken lightly and a difficult for one for many of us with chronic conditions. The future for us isn't always as clear cut as it may seem, sometimes our priority is simply in staying alive. So please don't assume we are selfish; we may be avoiding pregnancy for other reasons than simply boosting our bank balances. Although if the reason is purely financial, then again the decision is solely ours.

*

As we near the end of our adventure through a sickly world together, let's look forward. Although we must part, do not weep, for I will always be with you; if not in person then most certainly in spirit. (I've decanted my bodily fluids into a bottle of vodka for you). Often the best place to start when looking to your future is going back to your past. I don't mean literally, obviously; I'm not an idiot! (Unless by such times as this book is being read in my future and time travel is possible then yes, obviously I mean literally, what are YOU, an idiot?!)

What I mean by this is think back to your teenage self. What did the 16 year old you want out of life? – Then work on what your situation is now and adapt it to fit. I don't mean GIVE UP ON ALL OF YOUR CHILDHOOD DREAMS; I just mean try to establish if the things you once so badly wanted are still a part of you and work on a way to bring some of that enthusiasm and drive back that you once had but may have lost. For example aged 16 I wanted to be the next Salvador Dali. I was besotted with art and every hobby I had was a creative one; from making jewellery, painting, to trying to force some semblance of style onto my first boyfriend. Now, I still love art and occasionally as a hobby I will paint and create things for my loved ones. It's not my 'job' it's just a fun thing I do. But now I write. This is my main creative outlet and it allows me to cleanse my head of stress and anxiety, it's my happy go-to place and it makes me feel more productive than I did in all the years of secretly binning my exes' hideously ugly red fleece.

*

Although depending on when you 'got sick' if you're looking back to a past that was illness free, it can give you a bit of a skewed view of your former life. When I think back to my life pre-disease, it seems I'm wearing rose-tinted spectacles so tight they're almost superglued to my skull. Torturing yourself with perhaps not entirely accurate moments from your past can often be unhealthy and detrimental to your recovery. In my somewhat hazy memories of my pre-pain, 'healthy' life, my days seemed to be fit to bursting with fun. Dancing, drinking, romance, carefree abandon, performing 14hr shifts with as little as a 10minute break, never worrying about running out of toilet paper… the list goes on. However it can be very easy to focus on the good stuff in the past when things in the present might not feel particularly great.

Me, I've kept a diary since I was around 12 years old. When I take a trip down memory lane and read through my own pages it can be hard; in particular throughout the months leading up to my eventual diagnosis. It's painful to recall how… painful life was. If I read my 'sick' diaries now, I read about pain and suffering. But I also read about a woman who was growing and learning about her body and heart. Learning how to use her own mind, how to separate the wheat from the chaff in her social circles and how to treat those around her with empathy and kindness.

I read about a woman *becoming* a woman in every sense of the word, and worrying about perhaps not becoming the type of woman she, or others wanted her to be. About a woman who was completely and utterly pant-wettingly terrified about wat was happening to her body, and about losing herself and the people around her. I cried into my own pages and struggled to remember that this woman was me. I realised that I had felt incredibly alone in my suffering for a long time, and how happy I am now that I don't have to go through that loneliness and confusion ever again. As I read my own forgotten words I felt sorry for this woman and the weird longing to reach out and tell her it will get better. I want to tell her that people love her and won't desert her, and that eventually the pain will get easier to bear. That she will end up happy with a hilarious and handsome man who loves cats just as much as her, because miracles do happen.

The truth is, and it's not as disheartening as it may initially sound here, is that you often *can't* do everything you once did in living with chronic illness. OK, OK, so you CAN go for your goals and reach for the stars and achieve everything you set out to because you are amazing and capable of anything blah, blah, BLAH, but it may (and probably will) be harder than it would be for a normal person. That's OK. In fact it's kind of awesome, what a great testament to how strong you are that you are doing everything your peers are doing alongside battling health problems! But it's also OK if you can't. If you look back on your pre-sick life and find things have to be ruled out that were once a piece of cake, it's OK. Accept that you can be proud of taking a step back instead of torturing yourself for what you can't do. The main thing to remember is to simply remind yourself of what made and makes you happy and to focus on making that happen. Don't put obstacles in your way or decide that your illness will limit or put an end to certain activities, as that might not necessarily always be the case. Look for solutions don't compound problems.

*

It's imperative we value ourselves and our abilities. When life often seems like a constant 'fight' to 'conquer' an illness or disability, it can be incredibly disheartening when we feel we are outside of ourselves vainly trying to grasp at the last semblance of our hopes and dreams. Much like marriage, so I've heard.

Stop treating yourself as an afterthought – prioritise you and your mental health and well-being above all else. You may feel a partner, child, employer is more important but what better position to care for all of those people than from one where YOU feel calm, content and at peace with yourself and your choices?

You're already reading this book so I *know* you are capable of making good decisions.

*

CHAPS!

Well hello again ladz!

Thanks so much for heeding my invaluable advice and for sticking with me right 'til the end, I so admire your dedication!

*But listen, as our time together grows near I wondered, what of **our** future gents? Where do we go from here? What of our 10 year plan? Am I moving too fast? I'm moving too fast aren't I? It's just I like you so much, you feel the same way yes? YES? OK, OK I'll back off. Maybe you just need your space, right? A few days apart, let you sort your head out or whatever it is people say? That will surely help! It'll allow you to see things more clearly and realise you DO want to commit! I can wait! If I have to, I'll wait for you. You know I'll do whatever you ask!*

I'LL WAIT FORVER FOR YOU.

I'VE MADE A COAT OF YOUR EX WIVES SKIN I LOVE YOU. xo

Acknowledgements

This book is *for women,* and as you may or may not have established by now, I'm lucky enough to be one! Even luckier to know lots of them too! What a treat. There is a bountiful supply of amazing ladies in my life who make me happier than a wedding to Jon Hamm officiated by kittens in bow-ties.

In particular I'd like to mention Jen and Sam (and their beautiful daughters Sophie and Belle) who I'm lucky enough to call my friends and am honoured to have watched blossom into the incredible mothers they are today. They are bringing up girls who I know will be bright, independent, beautiful and hilarious women and I can't wait to see what they will undoubtedly achieve.

Most little girl's first insight into womanhood comes from their mother and I've been hashtag blessed to have an incredible one in my life. My Mum has taught me so much about kindness, love and empathy. She has instilled her values on me, encouraged me to LAUGH A LOT and love deeply. She never wanted me to settle for anything less than the best in all aspects of my life and although perhaps I haven't always, I still aim to make her proud every day.

This book is dedicated to my Grandmother Peggy who I adored and who made me laugh hysterically. She taught me the importance of love and forgiveness, friendship, and of living life to the full despite obstacles life may put in the way. Hope we get the chance to birdy-dance again one day.

Finally thank-you to all the women (and men) who have taken the time to read this book and I hope it's reminded you that you are never alone! I cherish you and I hope you continue to cherish yourselves everyday xo

OH and how could I forget? Thanks MEN! I know like the best condoms, I've gently ribbed you throughout this book, but I do truly and deeply love you. Despite the fact that the technology now exists to replace you in almost every conceivable way, from opening difficult jars to giving us self-made orgasms, at the end of the day nothing compares to the heat of a warm human male body by our side. Well maybe an electric blanket, or a heat-pad, but those things cost and men are (generally) free; we pay only in our continued low self-esteem, insecurity and crippling self-doubt! A bargain!

I jest, of COURSE. You're all ace. I have the best man in existence to share my mortgage and vagina with. Thanks James I love you xo

Printed in Great Britain
by Amazon